Tolerating abuse is not support.

If you wouldn't do it to a puppy don't do it to a human.

Abuse is abuse no matter the excuse.

The couples that make it are the ones that can
work together against the common enemy.

You can't do it for her and you can't do it alone.

PMDD isn't her fault but it is her responsibility.

Fundamentally PMDD is chemistry.
Will power and good intentions will only get you so far.

Nothing changes if nothing changes.

There's nothing but conflict in that conflict.

No talking about anything substantive during luteal.
Including luteal.

Unenforced boundaries are just suggestions.

Don't set yourself on fire to keep her warm.

Please put your own oxygen mask on first
before assisting others.

There's no eggshells but the ones she's laying down.

It's not her fault.
But if she's not doing everything in her power
to prevent it happening *again* ...
then it's her fault.

"What usually happens is that people take the
biggest breath they can and go down
—
and don't come back up again.
They can't flail and they can't yell.
You could miss it."

Claire McCarthy, MD, Harvard Medical School[1]

1 https://www.health.harvard.edu/blog/5-things-parents-need-know-drowning-2016080910114

The Last Desperate Flail

PMDD Through a Partner's Lens

Phew-ThatWasClose
and
Members of the PMDDpartners Subreddit

Flail Press

Published April 2026
Flail Press
Denver, Colorado

Written by Phew-ThatWasClose and
Members of the PMDDpartners subreddit

ISBN: 9798234045973
LCCN: 2026908508

PMDD lies.

Always.

To everyone.

Especially to her.

Table of Contents

Preface

When I got out of jail my family encouraged me to get some therapy to help process what happened. Years of trauma culminating in being arrested and spending a night in jail … some therapy made sense. But this was after the pandemic and everybody was depressed. Therapy appointments were months out. So everybody said to journal.

I hated journaling. Some people love it but for me it just reopens old wounds, rehashes the same complaints, and resurfaces the pain. I just end up feeling angry and depressed - again. For why? It felt like screaming into the void and the void didn't give a rat's ass. So I went to the PMDDpartners sub and screamed there.

At the partner's sub they understood. They knew why I stayed in the relationship as long as I did. They knew why the pain was so deep. They knew about the confusion, the fog, the baiting, the twisted logic, the whiplash, the dread, the guilt, the shame. They knew about it all. So I stayed.

I stayed for me. This was something I was doing for myself. Being there, reading posts, contributing comments, helped me process what happened. And if it also helped someone else, that was a nice bonus. By sharing my experience I could validate others and maybe help them avoid the mistakes I made. Journaling with purpose.

After a few months I noticed I was saying the same things over and over as new people showed up with essentially the same story and the same questions. I wrote the mod and asked if maybe the sub needed a wiki with an FAQ. He responded that that sounded like a great idea and would I do it? Gulp.

And so I became a mod and wrote an FAQ for the wiki. Then we had a wiki with an FAQ. Kinda puny. So I mapped out a structure for the wiki and asked the community to contribute. One guy said he'd contribute something about attachment styles but never followed through. I get it, everybody's busy.

It became my habit that if I found myself answering the same question, or giving the same advice, five or six times, I would create a new wiki page or write a post about it. Sometimes both. Those wiki pages became the "Best Practices" section. Those posts became the core posts I rely on to explain big ideas without hijacking the discussion too much.

I did that because it helped me. The sub is often repetitive as relationships with severe PMDD in the mix follow similar arcs. But the continuing discussion, new perspectives, different experiences, often lead me to think through issues I hadn't resolved. Sometimes issues I hadn't even considered. And the writing helped me process. Helped me nail down the thoughts.

Along the way I formalized the rules and started enforcing them. I reworked the icon and figured out how to put a nice banner in place. I added community highlights to the top of the sub and navigation to other resources in the right hand column. I generally tried to be of use, spruce up the place, and give something back.

Two years later and I've run out of things to write about. Not that there isn't more stuff - just that I've hit the limits of my experience and I'm really not qualified to talk about the more technical aspects. So I wondered if I had enough for a book and it kinda snowballed from there.

Introduction

PreMenstrual Dysphoric Disorder is a chronic, often *life threatening*, medical condition that gets worse over time. PMDD is not a hormone imbalance, but it sure looks like one. PMDD is an abnormal reaction to normal hormonal changes during the reproductive cycle. PMDD is a hormone driven neurological disorder.

Like PMS, and for many of the same reasons, it took decades for the medical community to recognize PMDD as a separate issue. In 1994 PMDD was listed in the DSM-IV in Appendix B: "Conditions for further study" and categorized as a "depressive disorder not otherwise specified." With the publication of the DSM-5 in 2013 PMDD was finally given it's own listing.

In the DSM-5 PMDD is defined as any five of a possible eleven symptoms and consequently it presents differently for everybody who has it. For many women the primary symptom is deep despair and Suicidal Ideation. Estimates are that over 30% of women with PMDD have attempted suicide. Not just thought about it - attempted it. Some have succeeded.

For some women with PMDD the primary symptoms are anxiety, tension, irritability, or anger. For some small percentage the primary symptom is Rage and the partners of those women are often caught in the cross hairs of that rage. Some of those partners find their way to the subreddit this book is based on.

There are few resources available for women with PMDD. Even fewer for the partners and caregivers. To my knowledge this is the second book on the topic. Aaron Kinghorn's "Hope" came out in the fall of 2024 and is an excellent resource for partners of women struggling with PMDD. Aaron speaks from decades of personal experience and has worked through tremendous difficulties in his relationship. I cannot recommend his book enough.

This book is a bit darker. The PMDDpartners sub is a small group of self selected partners who are well into the left hand tail of the bell curve. Well beyond despair, beyond anguish, beyond desperation even to the last last corner of the last last stronghold and *still* – there is hope – maybe.

There definitely is a lot of pain and a lot of anger. Since that anger is directed at women, one woman in particular, and has something to do with the reproductive cycle, it can be mistaken for misogyny. It's not. It's grief. Grief about what could have been and never was. Grief about the lost time and the shattered relationship. Grief about the partner lost to the disorder who briefly appears during follicular only to be swept away again.

And some of the anger you'll see in some of the posts and comments is the anger of the abused for their abuser. To be clear PMDD does not cause abuse. Rule #5 is pretty explicit about acknowledging that. But PMDD can cause Rage. And that Rage can be misdirected.

The idea that one would feel Rage so strongly for no reason beggars belief. It's absurd! There must be a reason. Look! There is my partner, my confidant, my love. The person who is supposed to make me happy. I am not happy. My partner is not doing their job!

Or maybe it's simpler than that. Maybe it's as simple as "She's mad, you're there." PMDD doesn't cause abuse, but it removes some guardrails, and it's often hard for a partner to recognize the abuse for what it is. "Pfffft. It's just hormones. She doesn't mean it. I'm tough, I can take it." All of that may be true. But it's cumulative and over time it degrades the relationship and destroys your soul.

The partners sub was the first place I identified my ex as "my abuser". It just kind of happened. At the time she was in menopause and the PMDD years were well behind us. I was just typing a comment and I typed that. I paused a second. I said "Oh." Then the bottom dropped out of the world and I was in freefall for about a half hour.

You'll often see references to "the other sub". That is the PMDD sub, the sub for the women who actually have the PMDD. Most of those women are very nice. Most of those women are not ragers. The suffering over there is real and raw and heartbreaking. I read that sub every day and comment if I feel I can help. Mostly I can't.

The intent is always to help. It is better for everyone – the partner, the PMDDer, and any kids – if the PMDD can be managed and the relationship healed. By the time folks get to the partner's sub that isn't always possible.

We always look out for the partner. Nobody else is going to. Partners often discover the sub after years, sometimes decades, of isolation, confusion, denigration, and self-doubt. The relief in suddenly finding you're not alone, and not the problem, is sometimes overwhelming. It was for me.

The point of turning the sub into a book is just to reach that small group that may not think to look for an online community. There are other books that are more hopeful, more constructive. This one is for the partners at the end of their rope, feeling trapped, feeling hopeless … yet … still. Somethings got to change.

There is some swearing.

The Rules

A community for the partners of people who suffer from PMDD. A place to ask for advice, or just to vent about your experience with PMDD. All opinions about PMDD will be allowed as long as you are kind to each other. This includes positive stories, advice, and even unfortunate situations where a PMDD relationship fails.

Rule #1: Be Nice - You can disagree without being disrespectful.

For example: If someone says your favorite youtuber is a charlatan and a snake oil salesman don't call them a "fuck face" and tell them to "Keep sucking the medical industry's nutsack". Is that oddly specific? Don't be that guy.

Rule #2: No Hate - No Misogyny, Misandry, Homophobia, Transphobia, etc.

For this sub we especially want to avoid directing any hate at "Women with PMDD". Most Women with PMDD are struggling mightily just to get through it day by day with minimal damage to themselves and those they love. If your partner is not an exemplar of that, that's unfortunate. Take a look at r/PMDD[2] to see hundreds of examples

Here's a really good one[3]
And here's thirty more.[4]

Rule #3: Don't Overgeneralize - Your sample space of one (1) is not statistically significant.

Your experience is unique. Every relationship is unique. Every woman is unique. You can speak from personal experience but you cannot predict how someone else's relationship will unfold.

We have a Negative Selection Bias here in that folks whose relationship with a partner with PMDD is *manageable* don't end up on the internet asking strangers for help and advice. Most of us stumbled across this forum only after things had gotten really bad. Nevertheless we are here looking for advice because we want to make things better. It's our last desperate flail.

If your relationship with your partner is profoundly negative that's horrible and I'm sorry you're experiencing that. Me too. But that is not inevitable and

---

2   http://www.reddit.com/r/PMDD
3   http://www.reddit.com/r/PMDD/comments/1cj05h1
4   http://www.reddit.com/r/PMDD/comments/1d9x2re

people come here seeking help, not prophecies of doom.

Rule #4: Don't say "They" - Every woman who suffers from PMDD is unique. Most of "them" don't do the thing you're saying "they" do.

A big problem with PMDD is that it covers a wide variety of symptoms and (probably) has a wide variety of causes. Women with PMDD uniquely suffer from different sets of symptoms to different degrees and respond differently to different treatments. So anytime you use the word "they" to lump all women with PMDD into a single category … you're wrong.

Try "some women with PMDD …" or "in my experience …" instead.

Rule #5: Abuse is Abuse - If your partner is abusive, that's Abuse, not PMDD. They may also have PMDD. Don't conflate the two.

One symptom of PMDD can be rage, sometimes "uncontrollable" rage. That rage should never be directed at another sentient being. Absolutely it should not be directed at a "partner". It's a partnership. We're in this together, as equals.

Most women with PMDD absolutely do everything they can to not take it out on their partner. Most women with PMDD recognize the irritability, or rage, as a symptom of the disorder and do what they can to redirect or deflect or isolate or whatever it takes to minimize the damage. Some, however, do not.

We get a lot of newcomers who have been tolerating the rage for months, sometimes years, and are at the end of their rope. As a community we need to call it what it is. It is not PMDD. It is not "because of" PMDD. It is Abuse[5] and it is not acceptable in any relationship ever. No way, No how, Never.

Tolerating abuse is not support. Her dumping on you every luteal just normalizes it. It's no fun for her either and it doesn't benefit anyone. It wears you down and it doesn't "get it out of her system". Rage begets rage in an upward spiral and saying it out loud reinforces the (false) notion that it's your fault.

It needs to be called out and addressed during the next follicular phase. You need a plan (p. 58) to avoid it next luteal. At least initially that plan should entail leaving the room, or the house, when/if it starts.

Rule #6: Cite Your Sources - If you assert something as scientific fact be

---

5   http://www.reddit.com/r/PMDDpartners/comments/1i1vjav

sure to include a URL for your source.

If you found out something new and want to share or have a question - that is awesome. Please include a link to your source. The answer to your question may be that your source is garbage. In that case we don't want everybody floundering about wondering.

A common method used by **Trolls** is to assert something controversial and then, when people object or question, be snide and patronizing and say stuff like "do your research." and "don't be lazy" and "every idiot knows this already" and "are you really that stupid?" and stuff like that. Trolls are weak little weasels who make themselves feel better by creating circumstances in which they can put others down. In this community we try to build each other up.

Don't be a Troll. Cite your sources. If you forget, and someone asks, respond with your source. Trolling will result in a ban.

Frequently Asked Questions

PMDD isn't her fault but it is her responsibility.

Fundamentally PMDD is chemistry.
Will power and good intentions will only get you so far.

Nothing changes if nothing changes.

Doctors have to know everything about everything
and consequently often miss something.
You only have to know everything about one thing.
Be the expert.

What is PMDD?

Premenstrual Dysphoric Disorder (PMDD) is caused by an abnormal reaction to the bodies normal hormonal changes during the menstrual cycle. Most notably an adverse reaction to increasing progesterone during the later "luteal" phase of the cycle. A more detailed explanation is in this post on the other sub[1].

There is no test for PMDD which is generally diagnosed by tracking symptoms[2] over several cycles and noting a periodic worsening of those symptoms. If the severity of the symptoms is not correlated with the cycle it's either not PMDD or not predominately PMDD. Treat the other thing first.

PMDD is not a hormonal imbalance. It is an adverse reaction to normal hormonal fluctuations. Many people get a hormone test first to rule out a hormone imbalance before seeking a PMDD diagnosis. That is a good idea, if your partner is able, as a hormone imbalance is a lot easier to manage.

PMDD can be exacerbated by a vitamin or mineral deficiency. That is also a much easier thing to manage so test for that. Most women are deficient in iron. 50% of people in general are deficient in Vitamin D especially in higher latitudes and/or winter. Some have reported complete relief by taking vitamin C daily. Don't mess around - test for everything.

---

1   http://www.reddit.com/r/PMDD/comments/1hucfm9
2   https://www.iapmd.org/shop/p/iapmd-pmds-symptom-tracker

What is a Cycle?

The menstrual cycle officially begins with the onset of menstrual flow, aka the period. The day menstruation begins is "day 1". This is the bodies recognition that pregnancy did not occur this cycle and it's time to reset the system. A decrease in progesterone signals the uterus to shed the lining it had prepared for the embryo. This typically takes about 5 days.

Follicules in the ovaries elongate in preparation for releasing an egg then all but one shrink back as the one swells and eventually does release the egg. This is called the follicular phase. This is the phase of the cycle when women with PMDD should feel at their best.

The release of the egg, ovulation, marks the beginning of the Luteal phase. This typically happens on day 14. Some women with PMDD experience a brief spike in symptoms at ovulation. Some women can feel the release. This is called mittelschmerz and can be painful.

Once the egg is released it begins to travel down the fallopian tube to the uterus. Increasing progesterone levels signal the uterus to begin creating a thick lining on the uterine wall for the egg/embryo to attach if necessary. It is the bodies reaction to the increasing progesterone that causes the symptoms associated with PMDD. This is the phase of the cycle when women with PMDD will feel at their worst.

For more detailed information see this article at the PMDD wiki[3] and this illustrated article at The Womens Health Network[4]

---

3   https://www.reddit.com/r/PMDD/wiki/index/cycle_basics/
4   http://www.womenshealthnetwork.com/pms-and-menstruation/your-menstrual-cycle-the-basics

How do I get my Partner Diagnosed?

The DSM-5 defines PMDD (p.268) as the presence of at least five of eleven potential symptoms, only during luteal, for two or more cycles. IAPMD[5] has a self screen for PMDD/PME[6] that can make the initial self diagnosis a little less confusing, but definitely follow up with a doctor who can prescribe treatment.

PMDD can be diagnosed by your ob/gyn, gp, psychiatrist, or other healthcare professionals typically by tracking symptoms for two or three cycles. You can save some time by starting now. Iapmd.org has a printable symptom tracker on their Tools and Resources[7] page along with printable information forms to fill out and take with you to the appointment.

Also on that page is a link to the Me v PMDD[8] app which includes a symptom tracker along with many other helpful functions. Another symptom tracker designed specifically for PMDD is Belle.[9] Belle also includes CBT support.

Note that even though PMDD is recognized in the DSM-5 (May 18, 2013) many medical professionals are skeptical/oblivious/ignorant. I asked on Reddit why that might be and was told Doctors are busy. So when she makes an appointment be sure to ask if the doctor has experience with PMDD. Your best course is to make yourself an expert so you can advocate for the treatment your partner needs. Read Everything.

More detailed information on getting a diagnosis is in the Best Practices (p.45) section of the wiki.

---

5   http://iapmd.org/
6   http://form.jotform.com/IAPMD/pmdd-self-screen
7   https://www.iapmd.org/shop/p/iapmd-premenstrual-disorders-pmd-infokit
8   http://mevpmdd.com/
9   http://bellehealth.co/

What Else Could It Be?

It could be a lot of things. PMDD is a diagnosis of last resort meaning it's not PMDD until everything else has been ruled out. A lot of things have symptoms that overlap with PMDD. Moreover many disorders can be mild, and not even recognized as present, but are then exacerbated during luteal giving the appearance of PMDD. Technically that is PME or Premenstrual Exacerbation.

For these reasons it is widely believed PMDD is misdiagnosed in 60% of women who have been diagnosed. This is bad because it means doctors, and patients, are treating the wrong thing. It works the other way too. Many women who have PMDD are initially diagnosed with something else and treatment is ineffective because the wrong thing is being treated. And, to further complicate things, people can have multiple disorders.

It may not be PMDD but it's definitely something. The best way to figure out what that something is is to pursue a diagnosis (p.45). PMDD is a diagnosis of exclusion which means systematically eliminating everything else it might be. Regardless of the outcome the process results in a pretty comprehensive picture of what is going on.

PMDD is often mistaken for Bipolar disorder. If your partner is Bipolar, but only half the month, they may have PMDD. Same, but less common, with Narcissism and Borderline.

The following are sometimes mistaken for PMDD. Many of these things are easier to treat.

- Hormone Imbalance
- Estrogen dominance
- High progesterone
- Histamine Intolerance
- Mast Cell Activation Syndrome
- Vitamin D Deficiency
- Bipolar disorder
- Borderline personality disorder
- General PMS
- Generalized Anxiety Disorder
- Major Depressive Disorder
- Attention Deficit Disorder
- Acid Reflux
- Sleep Apnia
- Iron Deficiency Anemia
- Iron Deficiency Without Anemia

These conditions can be exacerbated by the normal hormonal shifts during luteal making the problem appear to be PMDD when it is actually PME (Pre-Menstrual Exacerbation).

The PMDD sub has created a whole other sub about PME[10] which includes a dandy decision tree, based on the DSM-5 diagnostic criteria, to help distinguish it from PMDD.

---

10 https://www.reddit.com/r/PMEtheMRMD/

What if my Partner won't Accept the Diagnosis?

It can be a lot to take in and denial is fairly common. A life long condition that is a ton of work to mitigate … not fabulous. Especially if it has been undiagnosed for a long time and there is a history of conflict. Perhaps things could have been better if the diagnosis had come sooner. There's some grief involved in mourning the wasted time.

Approach that aspect of it delicately. It's often said "PMDD is not her fault but it is her responsibility." It's a medical condition, nobody's "fault". What if you found out she had a UTI that was making her cranky? Thank the heavens you now know what the issue is. Now you can address it together as a team. She needs your support now.

Where is the diagnosis coming from? If it's *just* your suspicion then you need to confirm. Iapmd.org[11] has a helpful self screen[12] she could take. Also see above for tips on how to get officially diagnosed (p.45).

If she still denies it's PMDD don't insist, just look to the symptoms. It doesn't matter what it is called. Many people with *these* symptoms find *these* things help. Just some basic vitamins and supplements can make a huge difference. That's not true in all cases but D, B12, Magnesium, and Iron are a good start. In my partners case that was sufficient and as a result she now denies she ever had PMDD. Doesn't matter. We got the symptoms under control after a decade of conflict. Call it whatever you want.

Indeed it might not be PMDD, or not just PMDD. Once you suspect it's an over-sensitivity to fluctuating progesterone levels maybe there is an over-sensitivity to other things as well. Try going gluten free for a week. Try eliminating sugar, caffeine, alcohol. Get some tests done. Iron levels are generally low in women. Other deficiencies may not be evident until the added stress of the luteal phase hits. It's worth checking everything.

As long as you are working together to mitigate the symptoms that's all that matters. Especially if there are kids you need to show by example how parents work together to solve problems and safe guard the family.

---

11 http://iapmd.org/
12 https://form.jotform.com/IAPMD/pmdd-self-screen

What are the Recommended Treatments?

If you haven't been formally diagnosed (p.45) do that. There is value in the process even if you're sure of the outcome. A *provisional* diagnosis can get you started on treatment while you confirm.

NB: Levonorgestrel is an extremely popular progestin used in many COCs, IUDs and Plan B. It is **not** recommended for PMDD because it has multiple properties that exacerbate PMDD symptoms even while controlling ovulation. Namely levonorgestrel has high androgenic and progestonic properties. The latter is especially problematic as it can cause *mood changes*, fatigue, *depression* and weight gain.

All hormonal IUDs contain levonorgestrel and consequently tend to make PMDD symptoms worse. Copper does nothing to regulate hormones so is useless for treating PMDD. The most popular Plan B, the one actually called "Plan B" is just a high dose of levonorgestrel and if you have PMDD it will cause a massive episode. The other option is **Ella** which contains ulipristal acetate and requires a prescription. For women with PMDD Ella is generally a lot less traumatic.

Yaz is the gold standard for PMDD because it contains drospirenone as its progestin which has *anti*-androgenic properties and low progestonic properties. Additionally drospirenone uniquely has antimineralocorticoid properties which help to limit water retention. Possibly less important but a nice bonus.

Zoely, Yaz, and Diane are specifically called out by RCOG. Zoely contains Nomegestrol Acetate and Diane contains Cyproterone Acetate. The chart near the top of the Birth Control page[13] on the other wiki is amazing. You should look up the progestin in whatever COC your doctor is pushing and find it in the chart.

Also **NB:** The recommendations do not specify, but the article does mention and other studies indicate, that **Mono**-phasic Combined Oral Contraception is best for PMDD. PMDD is an abnormal reaction to normal hormonal *changes*. **Tri**-phasic contraceptives change the mix every week.

Avoid COCs with "Tri" in the name. And as long as we're decoding "Lo" in the name means it's a low dose of hormones and "Fe" means the placebo contains iron. If you are treating PMDD you're not taking the placebo and probably need more supplemental iron than it would provide anyway. Get checked regularly and aim for ferritin levels around 100 ug/L to ensure sufficient stores.

---

13 https://www.reddit.com/r/PMDD/wiki/index/birth_control/

Royal College of Obstetricians and Gynaecologists (RCOG) Treatment Tiers below. The original piece with reference list and a case study <u>can be found here.</u>[14]

Staged Treatment of PMDD (Adapted from the RCOG 48 UK treatment guidelines)

Tier 1:
   1) Complementary Treatments – such as exercise, primrose oil, cognitive behavioral therapy, vitamin B6, magnesium.
   2) Combined Oral Contraceptive pill (COC) – taken continuously for 3 or more cycles (ie: without placebo pills). Newer generation COCs (Zoely, Yaz, Diane) are more effective than the older COCs, but differential depressive responses can occur in individual women.
   3) COC (continuous) + Antidepressant (<u>intermittent SSRI</u> (p.26) or SNRI or agomelatine)

Tier 2:
   4) COC + Estradiol patches (25 or 50 or 100 micrograms) + Antidepressant (intermittent SSRI or agomelatine)
   5) Estradiol patches (50 or 100 micrograms) + micronised progesterone (100 mg or 200 mg [day 17–28], orally or vaginally) + Antidepressant (intermittent SSRI or SNRI or agomelatine)
   6) Estradiol patches (100 micrograms) + micronised progesterone (100 mg or 200 mg [day 17–28], orally or vaginally) + Higher dose SSRIs or SNRIs continuously e.g. citalopram/escitalopram 20–40 mg, venlafaxine

Tier 3:
   7) GnRH analogues (Synarel) + add-back HRT (continuous combined estrogen + progesterone [e.g. 50–100 micrograms estradiol patches or 2–4 doses of estradiol gel combined with micronised progesterone 100 mg/day] or tibolone 2.5 mg/day

Tier 4:
   8) Surgery + HRT

---

14 http://www.vmiac.org.au/wp-content/uploads/HOW-TO-TREAT-PREMENSTRUAL-DYSPHORIC-DISORDER-copy-2.pdf

The American College of Obstetricians and Gynecologists (ACOG) has similar recommendations but in a more confusing format. The ACOG Clinical Practice Guideline No. 7[15] spells it all out, but is behind a paywall. Here is a copy that is not behind a paywall. A summary of the guideline[16] put out by The ObG Project is also confusing but more concise.

One of the mods at r/PMDD[17] distilled Guideline No.7 into a much more comprehensible infographic[18]. The image may be cropped when it comes up. Just click on it to see the full image. Then click on it again to zoom it big enough to read. This thing really should be poster sized on your Doctors wall. If you have the means have the copy center print it out and get your Doctor to put it up in their office.

Lifting from The ObG Project's summary - ACOG has only two categories:

Non-Surgery:
1) SSRI: low dose taken continuously or intermittently. Fast acting. (see details (p.26)) If used in adolescents, monitor for suicidal ideation.
2) Combined oral contraceptives - more effective than progesterone formulations.
3) Cognitive behavioral therapy - incorporating psychoeducation on anxiety triggers and coping mechanisms, including relaxation techniques, cognitive restructuring, and stress management strategies.
4) Routine exercise - Moderate exercise such as Aerobics, Yoga, Pilates.
5) Calcium supplementation - 1200 to 1000 mg/day.
6) Acupuncture[19].
7) NSAIDs - May benefit mood as well as pain symptoms.
8) Education.
9) GnRH agonists

Surgery:
10) Oophorectomy with or without hysterectomy - Prior Long-term GnRH agonist therapy is required. With or without estrogen add-back treatment.

---

15 http://journals.lww.com/greenjournal/fulltext/2023/12000/
    management_of_premenstrual_disorders__acog.34.aspx
16 http://www.obgproject.com/2023/12/27/acog-guideline-management-of-premenstrual-
    syndrome-and-premenstrual-dysphoric-disorder
17 http://www.reddit.com/r/PMDD
18 https://www.reddit.com/r/PMDD/comments/1b9qg75
19 http://www.reddit.com/r/PMDD/comments/1csqbaj

Notes:
* Screen for Suicidal Ideation.
* Many patients may benefit from a multimodal approach.
* Lifestyle and non-pharmacologic options include Exercise, Calcium, Acupuncture, NSAIDs, CBT.
* Vitex agnus castus - Chasteberry is an herbal supplement.
* In the adolescent population, symptoms of PMDD may be difficult to distinguish from the emotional variation found in normal development in this age group.

Low dose intermittent SSRIs: SSRIs (Prozac, Celexa, Zoloft, etc.) are generally used to treat depression. A therapeutic dose can take six weeks or more to *build up in your system* to be effective, can have unwanted side effects like low libido and lethargy, and can take months to ween off of when/if you decide to. If they work that's great. But if they don't work, or the side effects are unbearable, the whole miserable episode can take six months to a year to play out and leave you no better off. So they rightly they get a bad rap.

When used for PMDD the mechanism for how SSRIs work is different. "Low dose intermittent" means Doctors prescribe about a tenth to a fifth the therapeutic dose, and only during luteal so it *doesn't* build up in your system. There's no withdrawal but some cut the last dose in half anyway, just to taper off. And best of all it works *immediately* - if it's going to work. It's about the least medicated you can be and you'll see benefit right away.

See this post[20] for more information.
Scroll down to the middle for research sources[21].

See Also: Low Dose Intermittent SSRI Resources (p.26)

Perimenopause: For some Perimenopause turns into all luteal all the time and cranked up to 17. The Perimenopausal Estrogen Replacement Therapy study[22] (PERT) is a complex protocol for managing PMDD during perimenopause. One of the mods on the other sub wrote up this post[23] about her experience with the PERT protocol. Since peri can last 5-10 *years* it's well worth investigating.

For more information on perimenopause and PMDD check out the PMDD sub's wiki page[24].

---

20 http://www.reddit.com/r/PMDD/comments/1eipfdg
21 http://www.reddit.com/r/PMDD/comments/1eipfdg/comment/lgbq1dc
22 http://jamanetwork.com/journals/jamapsychiatry/fullarticle/2668205
23 http://www.reddit.com/r/PMDD/comments/1eo15yx
24 http://www.reddit.com/r/PMDD/wiki/index/perimeno

Low Dose Intermittent SSRI for PMDD — Resources

TLDR: Bunch of links to sciencey stuff about Low Dose Intermittent SSRIs for treating PMDD. In case your doctor doesn't know that's a thing.

SSRIs (or SNRI or agomelatine) work differently[25] for PMDD than they do for other disorders (depression, anxiety, ADHD). The mechanism for how they work[26] is different and consequently the treatment regimen is different. Many doctors *do not know this* and will want to treat PMDD the same way they treat other things. But for PMDD a much lower dose, during luteal only, is often more effective. Treating with a "therapeutic" dose everyday may be unnecessary and can lead to unnecessary complications like long term side effects, tachyphylaxis (tolerance), and serotonin syndrome (too much serotonin).

There are frequently posts on the other sub from women who *asked* for a low dose intermittent SSRI to treat their PMDD and were flat out told "That's not the way SSRIs work." Generally that is true, but for PMDD that is the way they work best.

A low dose intermittent SSRI is the *least medicated treatment* shown to be effective for PMDD, has no long term side effects (because you are not on it long term) will not lead to tachyphylaxis (for the same reason), and can work within hours, if it's going to work, so you don't waste a lot of time "trying" for months. The downside is you may have to advocate for yourself and educate your doctor. Here we have collected the resources you need to do that. You can just point your doctor here or, more impressively, print everything out and take it with you to your appointment. It's really hard to argue with someone who is waving a fistful of paper in your face.

If you are already on an SSRI for something else and it is *not* working for your PMDD the recommendation is to take a little more during luteal. This is called hybrid or semi-continuous dosing. One theory is that your regular dose is spoken for, your body expects it and takes it up immediately, and your PMDD needs it's own little bit. Effectively it's intermittent dosing on top of therapeutic dosing.

---

25 http://www.reddit.com/r/Psychiatry/comments/17ji14g
26 http://www.reddit.com/r/PMDDpartners/comments/1frjwfi

(Editor's note: The rest of this is a whole lot of links. If you have a print version of the book you're better off just going to the wiki page[27] when you have a chance and navigating from there rather than having a ton of footnotes cluttered at the bottom.)

One woman's experience.
And another.
And another.
And just one more.
And a whole bunch more.
And still more.
And still more.
And still more.

But do they work over the long term?

And some women who are especially sensitive to meds may need to even microdose their SSRI.

LDI SSRI is a first tier treatment recommended by both RCOG and ACOG.

- A clear readable listing of those treatment tiers is here.
- The original RCOG treatment tier appears in the RCOG 27 UK treatment guidelines.
- The original ACOG treatment tier appears in the ACOG Clinical Practice Guideline No. 7.
- A summary is published as ACOG Guideline: Management of Premenstrual Syndrome and Premenstrual Dysphoric Disorder

The original research was done in the 90's and 00's when PMDD was still not an official diagnosis.

- Steiner M, Korzekwa M, and Lamont J. et al. Intermittent fluoxetine dosing in the treatment of women with premenstrual dysphoria. Psychopharmacol Bull. 1997 33:771–774.
- Halbreich U, Smoller JW. Intermittent luteal phase sertraline treatment of dysphoric premenstrual syndrome. J Clin Psychiatry. 1997;58:399–402.
- Young SA, Hurt PH, and Benedek DM. et al. Treatment of premenstrual dysphoric disorder with sertraline during the luteal phase: a randomized, double-blind, placebo-controlled crossover trial. J Clin Psychiatry. 1998 59:76–80.
- Freeman EW, Rickels K, and Arredondo F. et al. Full- or half-

---

27 https://www.reddit.com/r/PMDDpartners/wiki/index/frequentlyaskedquestions/
recommendedtreatment/ldissriresources/

> cycle treatment of severe premenstrual syndrome with a serotonergic antidepressant. J Clin Psychopharmacol. 1999 19:3–8.

- Jermain DM, Preece CK, and Sykes RL. et al. Luteal phase sertraline treatment for premenstrual dysphoric disorder: results of a double-blind, placebo-controlled, crossover study. Arch Fam Med. 1999 8:328–332.
- Halbreich U, Bergeron R, and Yonkers KA. et al. Efficacy of intermittent, luteal phase sertraline treatment of premenstrual dysphoric disorder. Obstet Gynecol. 2002 100:1219–1229.

A more recent meta-analysis has highlighted that intermittent dosing is just as effective as continuous dosing for PMDD.

- Reilly TJ, Wallman P, Taylor D. et al. Intermittent selective serotonin reuptake inhibitors for premenstrual syndromes: A systematic review and meta-analysis of randomised trials Journal of Psychopharmacology, 2023 37(3):261-267.

And other studies have shown SSRIs can be effective for PMDD when used *as needed*.

- Yonkers KA, Kornstein SG, Gueorguieva R. et al. Symptom-Onset Dosing of Sertraline for the Treatment of Premenstrual Dysphoric Disorder: A Multi-Site, Double-Blind, Randomized, Placebo-Controlled Trial JAMA Psychiatry. 2015 Oct 72(10):1037–1044
- Steinberg EM, Cardoso GMP, Martinez PE, et al. Rapid Response to Fluoxetine in Women with Premenstrual Dysphoric Disorder Depress Anxiety. 2012 May 29(6):531–540

Other and more recent studies can be found by googling key words such as "low dose intermittent SSRI for PMDD"

The FDA has approved three SSRIs for treating PMDD. Those are Fluoxetine (Prozac), Sertraline (Zoloft), and Paroxetine (Paxil). Other SSRIs may also be of benefit off-label. Representative FDA labels are linked below.

FLUOXETINE- fluoxetine tablet, Torrent Pharmaceuticals Limited

SERTRALINE- sertraline tablet, film coated, Bryant Ranch Prepack

PAROXETINE- paroxetine hydrochloride hemihydrate tablet, film coated, extended release, Bryant Ranch Prepack

Studies show that continuous dosing is "just as effective" as intermittent or luteal only dosing. In general those studies lasted about three months. Three months is about exactly how long it takes for your body to get used to an SSRI and many women report their continuous SSRI stopped working for their PMDD after four months. That's my empirical impression from reading the r/PMDD sub for years and I am not a doctor so take that as you will.

Additionally studies show a *low* dose is effective for PMDD and generally the low dose studied was the lowest recommended dose for *other disorders*. But the way SSRIs work for PMDD is completely different to other disorders and many women report lower doses, even micro-doses, are effective. Again that is empirical but you might try tapering up (1/4, 1/2, 3/4, 1) your first cycle to see if you really need the whole thing. Or if you have bad short term side effects you might try cutting your dose in half to reduce side effects while keeping the benefits. Especially if you have been med sensitive in the past. But again, I am not a doctor.

Partner's Advice

We frequently say "Tolerating <u>abuse</u> (p.211) is not support." But what **is** support? **Ask** your partner what she needs. Talk about it during follicular but in general take as much off her plate as you can during luteal. What would you do if she had the flu? Do more. Of course you can't do anything while you're being yelled at so if she's yelling at you take that as a sign she wants to be left alone. Go get a froyo. Bring her back one.

When you talk to your partner about what they need during luteal write it down and make a plan. The plan should be as concrete, specific, and detailed as possible. Post it on the fridge. <u>There is a sample here</u> (p.69).

But some women with PMDD just won't. You can't do it for her and you can't do it alone. What are you to do? Here are some tips.

Go get a froyo, bring her back one.
Hard to stay mad at someone who brought you a froyo.

Turns out it's calming things that calm you down.

Whatever you do when you can't take it anymore …
do that right away.

From Baloneous_V

No.1 take a vacation from it during luteal. Figuratively and/or literally. No talking about it, no talking about your wishes, no really nothing. No vulnerability, no sharing, no progress, no growth. (This is the hardest part for me as a progressive person).

No. 2 Research empathetic assertiveness. Learn to draw boundaries (outside luteal) use the good times to stretch everything you don't get during luteal, and use the former to LEAVE before conflict during luteal... see 1.

No. 3 to get the former and a sense of control, instill a tracking means and method. If she won't, you will. If she doesn't like it that you do and she won't, do it as your secret mission. It is afterall with the intent to keep you together. You're not leaving her, or cheating. It's a sense of control for you to "know".... then you can act accordingly. That was my 2nd most need. A heads up and prep is worth everything. I still get surprised.

No. 4 the rest is learning what to give her and serve her when she needs it. You have to let go of the thought it's 50/50 during luteal. Plus you have to learn how to earn 50/50 balance outside of it... that's the hardest part bc it's never really balanced. See "boundaries" above. See "never speak of it" above. It is helping her, maybe, but you can never really point that out.

No. 5 seek like minded individuals and lean on them for advice so you don't feel alone (see this sub reddit)... aloneness is my hardest of all the hard. You can't share with your partner what affects you the most.

If all else fails, seek the advice of the first comment. Leave. You presumably don't have a marriage and kids, that's good. Seek yourself first. I am now my best and most trusted friend bc of this condition.

Find the silver lining and decide it's worth it, or not.

From MustyEssay

Here's some tips

1) Seek professional counseling if you can afford (someone that understands PMDD)
2) Take space for yourself during her luteal phase including sleeping in a different location if that's helpful.
3) Have important conversations outside of luteal phase
4) Know that your wife is probably feeling terrible about her behavior and very guilty.
5) Listen to some podcast episodes of PMDD stories, you'll hear repeating themes that relate.

The original comment on the sub.[1]

---

1   https://www.reddit.com/r/PMDDpartners/comments/1bbdfn7/comment/kudof9r/

Also from MustyEssay

Here's some things that have been helpful to name a few.

1. Knowing the cycle - when is luteal phase. If I don't know, it'll catch me off guard.

2. Check in on mood - Best thing for us has been a whiteboard marker on the bathroom mirror that she marks down her mood out of 10 each day. It gives me a chance to see when things are declining for her and being more proactive with what she needs. It's amazing how connected I feel to her with that number, she doesn't even need to say a word to me.

3. Know what she needs during the different phases (space, touch, silence, conversation, chocolate, snacks, extra sleep etc)

4. Accept both your needs, and support them. Accepting my needs/boundaries and sticking to them.

5. Know the triggers - ex messy house during luteal = no bueno. So we make sure to clean up days leading in to luteal.

6. Take advantage of the window where things are good. Like going out for dates, spending time together, being more physical. etc.

The original comment on the sub.[2]

---

2   https://www.reddit.com/r/PMDDpartners/comments/18a50ly/comment/kudmb4q

From IndelibleScrapyard429

A few strategies we have had to employ:

1) **Have a plan**. Recognize the symptoms, acknowledge them for what they are, and implement the action plan. The plan is going to look different for everyone and you should have a couple different ones for different situations.

2) Once the bleeding has started and emotions are normalized have some good communication. Usually issues brought up during a PMDD attack are real annoyances but are amplified by %1000. Wait until you are both in a good place to address them.

3) Take responsibility. My wife is so good at this. I am much more willing to forgive when I see her putting everything she has got into managing this illness. She gives %110 so I KNOW that when she is freaking out that it is truly outside her control. She acknowledges that the things she says during attacks are abusive and inappropriate and apologizes without groveling and still maintaining compassion and respect for herself. I have to do the same. I work hard. I apologize. I forgive. It's hard. You can do hard things.

4) Build a strong relationship outside of the PMDD reality. Make the good times REALLY good because you're going to need to look towards them with faith that it'll return to that once the chemicals get flushed out of the old luteal noggin.

5) Educate yourselves. Read the science. Objectifying is a good step towards compartmentalizing.

6) It is critical for us to develop ourselves as individuals. Some degree of emotional independence is required. Interdependence is a spectrum but highly emotionally codependent relationships will struggle under PMDD.

7) Emotional management isn't about repression, its about regulation. I feel my emotions and own them, but ultimately I am the boss of them. Studying and practicing Stoic philosophy helps.

8) Grow up when it comes to the egos. This is required by both partners. This one is hard to give advice on. Humility is a skill that can be practiced but part of this one is getting in tune with (and having faith in) something bigger than yourself. This looks different for everyone. For me it was taking mushrooms and talking to my future kids in the spirit world. If that's too woo woo for you… I don't know… Go to church or something? Whatever you gotta do.

Hope this helped.

From OkContext5658

If you want to make it work with her then;

* Track her cycle so you know when the PMDD is starting, this way if she starts acting out you're mentally prepared for the changes in her behaviour.
* Schedule more time with friends, family and focus on your hobbies or work projects so your focus is on you and not her during that time frame.
* When she lashes out/gets personal, do your best to keep your energy consistent whilst letting her know you're not going to engage whilst she's experiencing PMDD but will be open to talking about it once she's out of the cycle if she still feels the same way (which she likely wont).
* Post PMDD she is likely to feel a lot of shame and guilt about the way she behaved so avoid being critical if you can.
* Once she is out of the luteal phase and no longer experiencing symptms of PMDD it is the best time to trouble shoot together about BOTH of your needs and boundaries because she will be in a place to discuss that with you.
* Give her and yourself plenty of time/space to yourselves whilst she is experiencing PMDD.
* Ensure she has a support network outside of you whether that friends and family or a therapist so that she's not relying solely on you because its not your responsibility to fix her.

If she is not actively working on herself and making the individual aspects of her life better like her work/social life, health and well being then PMDD will likely magnify any gaps she's feeling and she'll take it out on those closest to her (typically …. not the same for everyone).

She has to be committed to making positive steps to improve her life in and around PMDD otherwise you will just end up feeling drained and the love between you both will be slowly but surely replaced with resentment. Walk away if she is not actively making an effort with you.

The original comment at the sub.[3]

---

3   https://www.reddit.com/r/PMDDpartners/comments/1b8lg81

From Mugatu-Utagum

Mugatu-Utagum went all out. This is his <u>entire post</u>[4] from June 6, 2024

Symptoms of being a PMDD Partner and Strategies for Managing

This is all based off my experience, patterns I've seen over the last 11 years, and what I've learned from this sub: (I hope this helps anyone suffering, looking for validation, and searching for hope)

COMMON SYMPTOMS

1. Emotional Strain:

- Increased feelings of frustration, helplessness, and confusion.
- Emotional distress due to witnessing the suffering of their partner.

2. Communication Difficulties:

- Breakdowns in communication, leading to misunderstandings and conflicts.
- Difficulty in maintaining emotional connection and intimacy.

3. Stress and Anxiety:

- Heightened stress and anxiety related to anticipating PMDD episodes.
- Concerns about how to support their partner effectively.

4. Relationship Strain:

- Increased tension and conflict within the relationship.
- Periodic feelings of distance or disconnection from their partner.

5. Fatigue and Burnout:

- Emotional and physical exhaustion from providing continuous support.
- Feelings of being overwhelmed by the cyclical nature of the disorder.

6. Personal Impact:

- Impact on their own mental health, potentially leading to symptoms of depression or anxiety.

---

4   http://www.reddit.com/r/PMDDpartners/comments/1d9bg6e

- Changes in personal routines and social interactions to accommodate their partner's needs.

7. Guilt and Self-Blame:

- Feelings of guilt or self-blame for not being able to alleviate their partner's symptoms.
- Concerns about saying or doing the wrong thing during PMDD episodes.

8. Need for Support:

- Recognition of the need for their own support systems, such as therapy or support groups, to cope with the challenges of being a partner to someone with PMDD.

Understanding these experiences can help partners seek appropriate support and develop coping strategies, which can improve the well-being of both partners in the relationship.

The emotional and relational challenges associated with supporting a partner with PMDD can significantly impact a partner's self-esteem, self-confidence, and faith in their own abilities. Here are some considerations and suggestions for managing these feelings:

Impact on Self-Esteem and Self-Confidence:

Feeling Inadequate:

- Partners may feel they are not doing enough to support their loved one, leading to feelings of inadequacy and self-doubt.
- The cyclical nature of PMDD can make it seem like efforts to help are never enough, perpetuating a sense of failure.

1. Emotional Drain:

- The emotional toll of dealing with PMDD can lead to exhaustion, making it harder to engage in activities that typically boost self-esteem.
- Constant emotional ups and downs can erode a partner's sense of stability and self-worth.

2. Social Isolation:

- Partners may withdraw from social activities to support their loved one, leading to isolation and a diminished sense of self-worth.
- Lack of social support can exacerbate feelings of loneliness and low self-esteem.

3. Impact on Personal Goals:

- Partners might put their own goals and aspirations on hold, leading to frustration and a loss of confidence in their abilities.
- Sacrificing personal time and ambitions can lead to resentment and a diminished sense of accomplishment.

STRATEGIES FOR MANAGING THESE FEELINGS:

1. Seek Support:

- Therapy or Counseling: Individual therapy can help partners work through their emotions, rebuild self-esteem, and develop coping strategies.
- Support Groups: Joining a support group for partners of individuals with PMDD can provide a sense of community and understanding.

2. Maintain Personal Interests:

- Engage in Hobbies and Activities: Pursuing personal interests and hobbies can provide a sense of accomplishment and joy, helping to rebuild self-confidence.
- Set Personal Goals: Establishing and achieving personal goals, even small ones, can boost self-esteem and reinforce a sense of capability.

3. Open Communication:

- Express Feelings: Sharing feelings and concerns with their partner can foster mutual understanding and support.
- Seek Professional Guidance: Couples therapy can improve communication, helping both partners navigate the challenges of PMDD together.

4. Practice Self-Care:

- Prioritize Well-being: Ensuring adequate sleep, nutrition, and exercise can improve overall well-being and resilience.
- Mindfulness and Relaxation: Practices like mindfulness meditation, yoga, or relaxation exercises can reduce stress and improve emotional regulation.

5. Educate Yourself:

- Understand PMDD: Learning about PMDD and its effects can help partners feel more equipped to handle the challenges and reduce feelings of helplessness.
- Stay Informed: Keeping up with the latest research and treatment options can provide a sense of control and empowerment.

6. Set Boundaries:

- Healthy Boundaries: Establishing and maintaining healthy boundaries is crucial to prevent burnout and maintain personal well-being.
- Time for Self: Ensuring time for self-care and personal activities can help balance the demands of supporting a partner with PMDD.

Rebuilding self-esteem and self-confidence is a process that requires patience, support, and self-compassion. By taking proactive steps to care for themselves, partners can regain a sense of balance and well-being while continuing to support their loved one with PMDD.

The original post on the sub.[5]

---

5   https://www.reddit.com/r/PMDDpartners/comments/1d9bg6e

Best Practices

For partners of people suffering from PMDD. You wouldn't be here if you weren't trying to work on your relationship to improve your entire family's life. With that in mind please note when it is recommended that you "leave" that generally means leave the room or leave the house. Stop sharing the same physical space. Many people who suffer from PMDD also have abandonment issues so be sure to tell your partner you'll be back. Just taking a break is all.

Each relationship is different so "best" practices may not always be the best idea in your circumstances. Still these are the methods that seem to be most effective most of the time.

PMDD doesn't have triggers, only excuses.

She's mad, you're there, that's it.

There's no eggshells but the ones she's laying down.

It's not her fault - but if she's not doing everything in her power to prevent it happening *again* - then it's her fault.

Safety Plan

When I was arrested Child Protective Services was called in automatically. As part of their standard response they had us create a Safety Plan to make sure everybody understood what to do to prevent another crisis and what to do if another crisis happened anyway. The template they had was all about making sure guns, drugs, and alcohol stayed out of the house. Certainly you should do that if you haven't already. None of those things were an issue with us so CPS were at a bit of a loss.

PMDD is a serious medical condition that affects every member of the family and can lead to severe or hazardous consequences quite quickly. It is not hyperbolic to call a plan for dealing with PMDD a "safety plan". Still a person with PMDD may feel a bit uncomfortably singled out. Feel free to call yours an "action plan" or "The PMDD Plan" or something neutral like "George". Here we shall still call it a safety plan to stress its importance.

The single *most* important thing to include in your safety plan is an agreement not to talk about anything substantial during the luteal phase. Most everything else stems from that. How do you break off a conversation that is starting to spiral? If one partner needs to leave for a cooling off period where do they go? If someone needs to leave the house for a bit who is it? And where do they go? and when do they come back? If someone doesn't adhere to the plan what's plan B?

The rest of the safety plan is a detailed description of what each partner needs during luteal to feel safe and cared for. Generally this means the partner without PMDD takes on as many chores as possible to give the other partner space and grace to do self care. This part of the plan needs to be quite specific. "Do more chores" and "do self care" are not specific and that will trip you up when you do the wrong chores, or not enough chores, and the PMDD wants to pick a fight. Imagine she has the flu. How does that play out in your household. Write that down.

Put it on paper and review it often. After every luteal phase figure out what went wrong and adjust the plan accordingly. Add in new things to try as you become aware of them. Do your research so that you become aware of new things to try. If you have agreement and buy-in before the fact you are much more likely to succeed when the pressure is on.

Down at the bottom of their Tools & Resources[1] page iapmd.org has downloadable templates for both an "action plan"[2] and a "safety plan"[3]. There

---

1   https://www.iapmd.org/shop/p/free-iapmd-premenstrual-disorders-pmds-treatment-
    guidelines
2   https://www.iapmd.org/shop/p/free-iapmd-safety-plan
3   https://www.iapmd.org/shop/p/iapmd-pmdd-action-plan

is also an <u>example safety plan</u> on this wiki that demonstrates the kind of specificity partners on this sub tend to need.

Take a look and modify to fit your specific needs or just write down your own thing. But do write it down. It's not a contract. You're not going to sign it and hold each other to "the agreed upon terms" or whatever. That would be dumb. It's just to have multiple modalities (talking, listening, writing, reading), a reference in case you forget some details, and something to discuss and modify next cycle.

Journaling

Journaling serves several purposes the most important of which is to create a record of your partners cycle that can be used to initiate or confirm the diagnosis of PMDD. It doesn't have to be anything elaborate. Just the date and how the day went. If it was a good day you might write why - "Took Bobby to the park." If it was a bad day definitely write why. If you want a more detailed record consider the IAPMD symptom tracker[4].

If your partner is taking meds or supplements record if they took them that day. One symptom of pmdd can be brain fog so they may forget. Gently remind. It is also common for people to stop taking meds or supplements when they feel better. Check that isn't happening during the follicular phase. Recording it in your journal or log means you're paying attention and they can't later tell you it didn't work if they haven't even taken it. Additionally you can track if new meds or supplements have an affect. You take your meds too. We're all in this together.

You're not trying to scrutinize your partners behavior but you are trying to make sure you know what's going on with their cycle so there are no surprises. Record what day of the cycle it is. The first day of their period is day 1. Many PMDD sufferers report it's infuriating to yell at their partner and have their partner respond with "Oh, is it luteal now?" No matter when it is in their cycle they are now doubly annoyed. Just know so you don't have to ask and can take appropriate care. Some PMDD sufferers report their partner tells *them* when it's luteal.

Lastly a contemporaneous record is invaluable if worst comes to worst and you find yourself talking to the police or getting a divorce. Make sure your journal is safe and backed up.

---

4   https://www.iapmd.org/shop/p/iapmd-pmds-symptom-tracker

Getting Diagnosed

If you haven't already try the self screen[5] at IAMPD[6]. While you're there grab some symptom trackers[7] and an appointment sheet[8], and read their take[9] on getting a diagnosis. Also read what the PMDD sub has to say[10] about it, what Mind has to say[11] about it, and what The PMDD Project has to say[12] about it. Multiple perspectives is always a good idea.

For symptom tracking I like the paper trackers because filling them out creates a chart with an undeniable rise and fall of symptoms that is easy for doctors to see. If you prefer electronic the other sub has developed a spreadsheet that accomplishes the same thing but in color! Note that you cannot be treating (p.22) for PMDD while symptom tracking to diagnose PMDD. OTOH if you *are* treating the PMDD and *still* having symptoms that may be something to bring up with your doctor when you ask for a med eval or a step up in the treatment tiers.

Take a look at the diagnostic criteria (p.268) before you get started.

Finding a Doctor

PMDD Is an abnormal reaction to normal hormonal changes during the reproductive cycle. As such it sits in the intersection of psychology and gynecology. PMDD can be diagnosed by:

- Your Primary Care Physician or General Practitioner
- Your gynecologist
- Your psychiatrist
- Your therapist.

Note your therapist may not be able to prescribe but they can still give you a provisional diagnosis and send that to your PCP/GP. Similarly a Psychiatrist will not be able to rule out the more physical/physiological possibilities but a provisional diagnosis can get you started on treatment (p.22). The least medicated treatment is a low dose intermittent SSRI (p.26).

If you have a health care professional you especially like make an

---

5   https://form.jotform.com/IAPMD/pmdd-self-screen
6   https://iapmd.org/
7   https://www.iapmd.org/shop/p/iapmd-pmds-symptom-tracker
8   https://www.iapmd.org/shop/p/iapmd-appointment-sheet
9   https://www.iapmd.org/steps-to-diagnosis
10   https://www.reddit.com/r/PMDD/wiki/index/diagnosis
11   https://www.mind.org.uk/information-support/types-of-mental-health-problems/premenstrual-dysphoric-disorder-pmdd/getting-a-pmdd-diagnosis
12   https://thepmddproject.org/wp-content/uploads/2025/01/How-To-Diagnosis-Digital-03.pdf

appointment with them. If you're struggling to access healthcare due to long wait times make multiple appointments now and get on the wait lists for cancellations.

Too few doctors are knowledgeable about PMDD. *Ask* when you make your appointment. Just say "I think I have PMDD. Has the doctor treated women with PMDD before?" It will do you absolutely no good to wait months for an appointment only to have your concerns dismissed. Note also that some gynecologists focus on medical/surgical care, rather than female hormones or menstruation. It is wise to ask what their specialty is and what they regularly treat before booking an appointment.

Ultimately the type of doctor you see is less important than the extent of their knowledge and empathy. IAPMD has a Provider Directory that may have a listing in your area. That directory is a growing resource so if you find someone good please submit their information. (IAPMD is currently recovering from a security breach. The Provider Directory is currently off line and many resources are missing while they rebuild.)

Getting Started

PMDD is diagnosed by tracking symptoms for two or more cycles so print out the symptom trackers (p.299) and get started. Even if you have tracking in your phone already paper copies are going to be easier to show your doctor and the charts from IAPMD have a good layout for visualizing the cycle. If you already have your symptoms tracked in a journal or an app transfer what you have to the charts.

Just the tracking data is sufficient to get you a *provisional* diagnosis and started on treatment so long as you are not seeking anything radical.

Testing

PMDD is a diagnosis of exclusion. It's only PMDD if it's not anything else[13] so start excluding things that have similar symptoms. Ask to get blood tests for hormonal imbalance and vitamin and mineral deficiencies. Get those tests done now so you can talk about them at your appointment.

Testing for hormonal imbalance is typically a blood test around day 20 (for progestin and estrogen levels). To be thorough some providers do an additional test around day 3 (for estrogen, follicle-stimulating hormone (FSH) and lutenizing hormone (LH)). PMDD is *not* a hormonal imbalance so if you have PMDD your hormone levels will be normal. If your hormone levels are

---

13 https://www.reddit.com/r/PMDD/comments/1lisdgc

abnormal work with your doctor to fix that.

Testing for vitamin and mineral deficiencies is also a blood test. Most people are low on Vitamin D. Most women are low in Iron. Pay special attention to the ferritin level. Iron Deficiency Anemia (IDA) is shown by ferritin levels below 15 ug/L. But Iron Deficiency Without Anemia (IDWA)[14] presents a lot of the same symptoms as PMDD. Try to get ferritin levels up to around 100 ug/L. Women lose a lot of iron every cycle so having sufficient reserves can be critical, but not too much. Ferritin levels above 200 ug/L are dangerous and above 300 ug/l are toxic.

And as long as they are taking blood get ALL the labs just to be safe. A1c, lipids, micro-nutrients, CBC, metabolic. PMDD is a diagnosis of exclusion so EVERYTHING[15] else needs to be ruled out.

- Hemoglobin A1c tests blood sugar. High A1c means you're pre-diabetic or diabetic. Low A1c can indicate hypoglycemia. Symptoms of Hypoglycemia include fatigue, dizziness, headache, irritability, rapid heartbeat, difficulty concentrating, and anxiety.
- A lipid panel tests for various kids of lipids (fats). Low cholesterol is rare but symptoms can include fatigue, joint pain, and muscle weakness. Symptoms of high cholesterol can include stroke, heart attack and death.
- Micro-nutrients include all the vitamins and minerals you need a little bit of. Vitamin D and iron, mentioned above, are the main ones.
- In addition to Vitamin D make sure you have enough A, B complex, C, and K. Vitamin B especially helps with making red blood cells so symptoms of a deficiency can be similar to IDA and PMDD. Symptoms of vitamin B deficiency include irritability, confusion, poor judgment, lack of coordination, fatigue, and depression.
- In addition to iron make sure you have enough magnesium, zinc, potassium, and calcium. Extra calcium is explicitly recommended by RCOG for women with PMDD but excess calcium can interfere with the absorption of iron and magnesium so you may wish to space those three out. Magnesium helps with sleep so many people take that at bedtime.
- A Complete Blood Count (CBC) measures the type and quantity of cells in the blood. A CBC is a pretty basic front line test to check for things like anemia and infection.
- A Metabolic blood panel measures a variety of different substances in your blood, such as glucose, electrolytes, and

---

14 https://www.reddit.com/r/PMDD/comments/1g13ask
15 https://www.reddit.com/r/PMDD/comments/1l8wbhp

proteins, that indicate your overall metabolic health. Abnormal levels can indicate things like diabetes, nutritional deficiencies, dehydration, as well as possible kidney or liver issues.

Treatment

First tier treatment (p.22), Item 1, is:

Complementary Treatments – such as exercise, primrose oil, cognitive behavioral therapy, vitamin B6, magnesium.

Start that now. Can't hurt might help. Add in C, B12, Zinc, Potassium, and especially Calcium. Sounds like just a good women's multivitamin or prenatal vitamin but some minerals inhibit the absorption of others. Specifically take magnesium separately as the magnesium in your multi is likely ineffective. Magnesium glycinate helps with sleep so maybe take that at bedtime.

While you are waiting read everything. As mentioned above many doctors have too little knowledge about PMDD so you may need to be the expert. Know what the treatment options (p.22) are and know what you want going in. The least medicated treatment recommended by both RCOG and ACOG is a low dose of an SSRI during luteal only (p.26). That is completely different to how SSRIs are used for other disorders and many doctors do not know that so, again, you may need to be the expert.

Here is an app developed for tracking PMDD symptoms[16]
Here is another app for PMDD[17] that includes CBT support.
Here is a printable symptom tracker[18] to fill out.
Here is a different printable symptom tracker[19].

---

16 https://mevpmdd.com/
17 https://bellehealth.co/
18 https://www.iapmd.org/shop/p/iapmd-pmds-symptom-tracker
19 https://www.stjoes.ca/hospital-services/mental-health-addiction-services/mental-health-services/women-s-health-concerns-clinic/pmdd-chart.pdf

Follicular

Follicular is the first half of the cycle. Her period begins (day 1), progesterone levels have dropped, and she should be feeling like her normal self again. Take a few days to recover if luteal was tough this cycle. But then start preparing for the next luteal phase. It's coming in two weeks.

Discuss any issues that came up but were put off. Verify that those issues were only issues because of the PMDD. If you tried something new discuss how effective it was or wasn't. If the safety plan (p.58) needs to be tweaked do that now. Keep what works, replace what doesn't and add new ideas as they come up. If the plan went off the rails at some point discuss a new strategy to stay on track next time.

But don't *just* prepare for the next Luteal. Follicular is when she's feeling her best. This is the woman you fell in love with. Follicular is the time to strengthen the relationship and create the good memories to sustain you. Go out with friends, have friends over, have date night, take a weekend trip, binge watch Upstart Crow. Whatever the two of you enjoy together - do a lot of that.

Luteal

Luteal is the second half of the cycle. The luteal phase begins with ovulation (day 14) and progesterone levels increase as the uterus prepares for implantation of the embryo. Ovulation can trigger an almost instant onset of PMDD symptoms for some. For other's it can be just a slow building of symptoms through luteal. In her 2003 book The PMDD Phenomenon Diana Dell identifies 5 distinct patterns of PMDD. Get to know your partners pattern.

If your consistent efforts during the rest of the cycle are effective the luteal phase may be manageable. Otherwise it's time to hunker down and get through it.

Now is when your partner is really suffering so as their partner you need to step up and provide what support you can. Extra chores, comfort food, distracting shows, take care of the kids, do more of the driving, etc. Basically giving your partner extra time and space to do what they need to do to get through a difficult time

Many PMDD sufferers report symptoms like extreme exhaustion, depression, irritability, and suicidal ideation, as well as the physical symptoms of bloating, cramps, joint pain, and headache. Whatever your partners particular mix is they are doing their best and need your support, Be attentive, but don't hover.

The most damaging symptom during luteal is the rage. Many folks with PMDD report wanting to break up with their SO every cycle during the luteal phase. Do not have any serious discussions about your relationship during this part of the cycle.

Do not have arguments of any kind during the luteal phase. PMDD can sometimes cause extreme anger about trivialities. It does not help to point out that the concern is trivial. It does not help to apologize (p.117) for an imagined infraction. When confronted with an angry partner who appears irrational there is no "talking them down." Engaging just adds fuel to the fire.

Many people report their partners with PMDD will try to bait them into unproductive, but escalating, arguments. As soon as you become aware you are being pulled into such an argument back off. If you find yourself becoming angry, and you know or suspect it is caused by the PMDD, take a deep cleansing breathe and tell your partner you will talk to them about it next week.

If they insist on talking now, you need to hold firm. This is a boundary you already set in your safety plan. These types of discussions can spiral out of control quickly - so it is a safety issue. Don't say that, obviously, but hold your boundary. <u>If you must leave then leave</u> (p.107). Tell your partner you will be back but for now you both need some space.

Tolerating abuse is not support. Nobody benefits. Leave the instant it starts. She can't trash you if you're not there. She just feels rage. If you're there she'll rage at you. Then she'll have rage AND regret. Take a walk, go work out, have a froyo, bring her back one.

Leaving can present it's own challenges. In extreme cases your partner may try to prevent you from leaving. Do not get physical. Leave by another door. If you are trapped, or can't leave for some reason, you may now have an opportunity to practice greyrocking. Remember the point of greyrocking is to be boring. Do not engage. You will talk about all this next week when you review what went wrong with the safety plan. For now just get through with minimal damage.

Cycle

No surprises - Put her cycle on the calendar and/or have a shared period app. Make colored laminated cards to leave around the house as reminders. Make a fire danger spinner and put it on the fridge. Some women wear a special piece of clothing or jewelry during luteal to remind *themselves* their thinking may be hijacked. One woman writes her cycle day number on the bathroom mirror. Make sure everybody knows so nobody has to ask. The only thing worse than being cranky because of PMDD and having some yahoo ask if you're cranky because of PMDD is being cranky for legitimate cranky-making reasons and having some yahoo say "Is it luteal already?"

Arguing

The single worst symptom of PMDD is the Rage, and that leads to arguing. Most people who end up on reddit seeking advice from strangers about PMDD are here because they've experienced the rage first hand and want it to stop. Arguments fueled by PMDD are the worst.

Don't participate.

That's it. That's the secret and the key. Nancy Reagan said it best.

Just say "No."

No arguing during luteal. If you want to argue, <u>leave</u> (p.107).

Eggshells

Can't do anything right? Feel like you're walking on eggshells? Trying so so hard not to even breath wrong because she will go off? Relax. You can't do anything right so what are you worried about? <u>As one member commented</u>[20]:

Infoseek456 - May 19, 2024

Starve the fire of oxygen. Don't engage the crazy illogical statements and accusations. Draw your line in the sand when she starts getting like that, and walk away.

This is easier said than done, but much easier to do when you KNOW what time it is. It's somehow always still a surprise, but when you are waiting for it, it's easier to act accordingly.

You don't need to walk on eggshells- because you aren't the trigger. It's not (within reason) what you say or do that causes this- she's going to find something no matter what. So stop putting all your energy in yo worrying about what you're doing/not doing, because it doesn't matter.

You can't reason with crazy- a misunderstanding of facts is not what's behind the outburst. So save your breath.

They will find all kinds of ways to twist it around to you, and rail on you for suggesting it's them. But, if you leave it alone, it goes away. Because there is no actual problem in the first place.

"I'm not having this conversation right now." "If you really want to talk about this, we will. In 10 days we can sit down and talk as much as you want about this. I will not engage in this conversation now."

Repeat that a few times. And if you have to, walk away. Go for a walk. Tell them "ok, I'm going to walk away now, or I'm going for a walk I'll be back in [x] minutes.

Don't respond to the verbal assault that will likely come your way as you calmly and unemotionally disengage from whatever crazy conspiracy/accusation/name calling/blame game she's trying to start up, and go do what you said you would.

When you come back- don't re-engage. Don't bring it up. Don't act mad. Just continue on with your day and most likely it's over. At least this incident is. Because they've already forgotten about it, because there was nothing there

---

20 http://www.reddit.com/r/PMDDpartners/comments/1ct1kel/comment/l4rvwqx

in the first place. They know they're not right, so you'll either get an apology (good luck) or someone acting like nothing ever happened.

But if you stay and defend and try to reason, etc- it will just turn in to a bigger and bigger fight. You will get more and more frustrated, and they will turn the fight into justification to get more and more mad/hurtful and stay that way for longer.

Don't engage. Starve the fire of oxygen. And breathe, knowing that just as quick as that flip turns on, it turns off in another week. Does wonders for your own mental health.

Finding the Exit

To be clear: Most women with PMDD *do not* experience rage as a symptom. But if you're here …

You've had the talk during Follicular. She refuses to acknowledge there's an issue, she refuses to seek a <u>diagnosis</u> (p.18) or <u>treatment</u> (p.22), she's adamant that you're the problem, she wails that she's tried everything <u>(really? everything?)</u> (p.284) or just deflects and accuses you of not being "man enough" to handle her. Now *your* health is suffering. You are not equipped or trained to handle this sort of thing. You tried your best. Sure you made some mistakes but overall you did an amazing job in an impossible situation. But you can't do it alone and if you're getting no cooperation from her … Time to leave.

If you have no entanglements (shared property, finances, lease, etc.) just leave. Block her if you have to so you don't get sucked back in. If you do get sucked back in just know that it takes an average of seven tries for abuse victims to leave their abuser, and try again. If you do have entanglements sort that as best you can, but quickly. Once you've decided to leave every day is precious and every day is dangerous. Until you are physically separated every interaction can be turned against you. So GTFO and if that means abandoning your record collection count yourself lucky.

Many women do not have PMDD until after the birth of a child. Pregnancy and childbirth is a significant hormonal event that shakes up the entire reproductive system. In many cases postpartum depression segues into PMDD and it just becomes the new normal. In some cases PMDD doesn't appear until after the second or third child. It can be an intensely confusing time for new parents. Regardless there's now a child, or multiple children, in the mix. That is a significant entanglement that complicates leaving a hundredfold.

If you are thinking about staying "for the sake of the children" <u>think again</u> (p. 273). Most women with PMDD will *not* direct it at their kids but the kids still see it, and hear it, when it's directed at you. I stayed because I thought the kids needed two parents. I came to realize they needed two *functional* parents and I was not that. My kids barely knew me and were growing up an anxious mess, like their mother, and her mother. I left so I could use my part of the shared custody to show them a better way.

Most lawyers will give you an initial consult for free. Talk to five. Be concise in describing your situation as you are there to get information, not to vent. Maybe write down a concise paragraph before the meeting. Have your questions ready. In the US laws vary by state. In Europe laws vary by country. Maternal bias is real everywhere because most domestic violence is man->woman. If you are making a case based on the abuse you have experienced, and fear will continue, expect an uphill battle and prepare accordingly.

The Arbiter in my divorce, a judge with 30 years experience, and a woman, *could not conceive of* The Man being the oppressed one in the relationship and dismissed my side of the story as *entirely* false. That's not me being dramatic or a sore loser. She wrote that in the divorce decree. Our PRE, also a woman, was equally biased.

We hadn't even heard of PMDD at the time of the divorce. We didn't even know it was a thing until two years after the divorce was finalized. At the time I didn't want to be a misogynist ass so I didn't bring gender up. I should have. Maternal bias is real. Opt for a male Judge, Arbiter, Lawyer, PRE, CFI, etc. if you have a choice.

Depending on your specific situation questions for the lawyer may include:

 What do I need to document to prove the abuse?
 What do I need to document to prove there's a mental health issue at the core of all this?
 Are written narratives of events useful, or just dismissed as biased?
 I've heard contemporaneous records count as evidence. Is that true in this instance
 I didn't write it down at the time. Is it useful to write it down now?
 Is audio or video recording useful? allowed?
 She is undiagnosed, but I strongly suspect PMDD. How can I get her mental health issues front and center?
 She is diagnosed, but refuses treatment, how big a deal is that?
 If full custody (for me) is not possible can we ask the court put her parenting time during Follicular?

If you fear your PMDDer will take it out on the children have all your evidence ready and file for full custody. I found out the hard way that in my state an *emergency* motion takes 14 days. That means nobody even looks at it for 13 days. My motion was denied because the emergency had passed by the time anyone looked at it so timing may be paramount. Maybe ask your lawyer if you can keep the kids and get a temporary restraining order on her and how does all that work

Making a Plan

I wrote a plan. Then I started collecting them. Whenever I saw a good one I asked the author if I could include it in the wiki. You'll see some themes.

Eventually I stumbled back to Llama's post and realized "my" plan is just a clone of his so credit where credit is due. Both are included here along with five from the other sub.

IAPMD.org has a sample "safety plan"[1] and a sample "action plan"[2] on their Tools & Resources[3] page. Both are more fill-in-the-blank type forms. You may like that better so take a look.

Luteal is no time to be asking questions.

No talking about anything substantive during luteal.
Including luteal.

Luteal is a lot less chaotic if it's scripted.

It seems weird because it is.
Everybody just does their thing and meet up on the other side.
Review and revise every follicular.

---

1   https://www.iapmd.org/shop/p/free-iapmd-safety-plan
2   https://www.iapmd.org/shop/p/iapmd-pmdd-action-plan
3   https://www.iapmd.org/shop/p/free-iapmd-premenstrual-disorders-pmds-treatment-guidelines

You need a Plan.

Phew-ThatWasClose - October 1, 2024

I see a lot of posts and comments on the other sub about how the boyfriend or the husband or the SO isn't supportive enough. Having been that husband I bristle a bit. Truth is some SOs are assholes but most are struggling just as much as she is. And "supportive enough" is a trigger phrase for me because "support" is a moving target and there's no such thing as "enough".

In my experience "I need your support." really means "Make me happy." When that doesn't happen it must be because I'm doing it wrong, or doing the wrong thing, or not doing enough. But we just can't. The disorder is making her miserable and the best we can do is create space so she can ride it out. We can provide support, but we can't make her happy.

So on both subs I advise folks to make a plan during follicular. The plan needs to be as concrete, and specific, and detailed as you can make it because luteal is no time to be asking questions. It needs to be written down so nobody forgets anything. And it needs to be posted on the fridge.

I admit to being a bit of a fraud as I never had a plan. By the time we got the diagnosis the damage was done and the need had passed. When I needed it I couldn't have written it anyway because I could barely string two sentences together. "Please Stop" was my mantra for years and if I had written a plan that's what it would have been. Reams of it.

Now, obviously, I can string two sentences together. So <u>I wrote a plan</u> (p. 69) hoping it might help someone else.

> QuercusSambucus
> Your link to the plan doesn't work for me.
>
>> iaamanthony
>> Same.
>>
>> GetTheLead_Out
>> Getting the page not found feels a little symbolic:) I'm joking, of course!!
>>
>> Plan not found, plan made and forgotten, no plan to be had. It's all seen here and at r/pmdd[4] daily.

---

4   http://reddit.com/r/pmdd

Thanks, as always, to phew for putting in work so hopefully others can suffer less and maybe stay together .

> Phew-ThatWasClose OP W
> What's that saying? How do you make God laugh?

>> QuercusSambucus
>> Mike, Tyson says everyone has a plan until they get punched in the face

>>> GetTheLead_Out
>>> And if anyone knows something about being punched repeatedly…

>>>> miliefisathand
>>>> i fucking felt this so hard. been feeling the punches ive been lectured constantly to roll over. ill roll over when im dead lol which is what she wants i think.

> Phew-ThatWasClose OP
> Thanks for pointing that out. Should be fixed. :(

GetTheLead_Out
Love the go bag idea! So wise.

And I want to highlight the not supervising of the tasks that someone is helping you with. This is important! If someone (partner) is helping with laundry, dishes, go on to bed or for that walk. The supervision just opens up discussion, and potential trouble.

> Phew-ThatWasClose OP
> Laundry and dishes are literally the easiest frickin things. That my partner made such a big deal about it, and refused to write down what she wanted done, was what clued me in that it wasn't about any particular thing. It was about control and subjugation.
>
> Her anxiety caused her to have control issues and her control issues caused her to denigrate everything in an effort to maintain the power up position.
>
> Hmmmmm. I'm an idiot. There was never a scintilla of a chance of a

possibility of a "partnership".

Good talk. Thanks. :)

GetTheLead_Out
Haha I'm really, really, really bad. I basically have to leave the room when anyone is doing dishes. One time, I silently turned the water off while my friend was washing her face, because she was scrubbing with it running. I said "tell me when you want it back on" and hovered over her. I have an intense water wasting trigger. She laughed and accepts my psychotic nature.

Point is. I am your wife. Unfortunately. But my ex divorced me pre hard core pmdd (but I have a feeling pmdd played a part, I just wasn't aware). Fortunately I date a bachelor who doesn't need to see me frequently. But I can't stand how he does dishes!!! I bite my tongue til it bleeds though.

Laundry, cooking, dishes, all of it is so hard for me to witness. Everyone does it wrong 😄. My college boyfriend (who was generally happy to be my doormat) told me point blank he wouldn't cook with me anymore if I didn't shape up. That cued me to how horrible I am. But it's still hard.

I'm not proud! And I do bite my tongue constantly now. But I wonder if lots of us pmdd ladies have this controlling nature streak to attempt to reduce our own vague anxiety. It sounds utterly stupid to say that for me listening to water running while someone is doing dishes puts me into intense physical discomfort and mental anguish. And that generally I just have to leave the room, hopefully somewhere not in ear shot. But it does.

You had kids. I think if you didn't fight (even if delusional) that would suck.

GetTheLead_Out
I don't know where you'd add it- but avoiding hunger, avoiding skipped meals. You talked about eating enough and healthy, but I find that particularly if someone is trying to lose weight, or generally come from a history of restriction (nearly every woman), sometimes skipping meals feels like a virtue. And sometimes refusing to eat can happen.

Or maybe don't add it. But sharing my insight. It's my 1 day to day item that I have to focus on.

Phew-ThatWasClose OP
Is that follicular as well? Like don't eat less, eat better ... kind of deal?

GetTheLead_Out
Sorry- in luteal don't go hungry

So in follicular sometimes I'll do light Intermittent fasting/push hunger. It's no big deal (still 5 lbs to go to get back to healthy weight, lost ~40 lbs a couple years ago).

In luteal, I can't let myself get hungry. So I keep diet style stuff to my period week and the week after. Day 14-28 I don't skip meals, and if I get hungry, I eat.

Yesterday I knew I'd be taking my niece and nephew to in n out in a couple hours and eat a full meal, but I was starving. So I ate 4 eggs with nothing else, scrambled. Then had my meal around 3:30, and was done for the day. This is luteal. If I would have been hungry at night, I would have eaten. In follicular , I'd maybe call it an Intermittent fasting day, and tolerated a little hunger.

Also, don't drive hungry, don't have conversations hungry (even via text). If i need to talk to someone, I eat first, if it's that time.

This is just me. But everyone will have a profile. Keeping a snack in the purse is wise.

Phew-ThatWasClose OP
Added a bullet to stress that point. Thanks.

GetTheLead_Out
Thanks!

Pristine_Motor_8699
'Keeping a snack in the purse is wise' Absolutely! I only figured this out recently. During follicular I can go five/six hours between meals no problem, but not during luteal. I try to have a reasonably healthy snack every three hours or so and I have noticed I am a lot less crabby.

GetTheLead_Out
If I start to feel myself feeling crazy, agitated, angry, first order

or business is to eat unless I ate like less than an hour ago.

I find the luteal hunger isn't logical. I could have eaten 2 hours before and start to get all agitated and hungry. In those instances I try to eat real food if at all possible (vs junk), but definitely eat again.

Unfortunately I think it can take years for a woman to accept that this is a non negotiable. For me it took me years to make the connection. And! If someone struggles with Interoception from being ND, detecting hunger is hard. But if you're agitated, headache, angry, sad, etc et. Try eating.

Pristine_Motor_8699
I totally agree. It's such a shame that it's so easy to get into the habit of ignoring what our bodies are telling us.

SaltVictory8301
This a great post. I'm in the no plan casualty section. This forum has been a great outlet since to see that I wasn't as alone as I felt at the time, and there are many other people trying their best but can't hack it without a clear strategy and plan. I'm not first hand dealing with PMDD anymore but trying to support the people who are is important.

FarReaction
Thanks, Phew, for making this plan. It looks great to me.

I don't think there's any way my wife would go along with Rule 1, even if we discuss it during follicular. She's been diagnosed with PMDD but still doesn't seem to see it being at the root of these horrible conflicts. We are doing couples counseling and I plan to bring up something like this at our next appointment.

To her, it feels severely emotionally disconnecting and triggers some kind of abandonment rage if I suggest we should put off a discussion, even just until the morning.

To me, it feels like I'm a punching bag on the end of a one-way stream of venting, anxiety, and rage. I try to empathize, validate, and grey rock, but I can only take so much of it, especially when I am drained from doing most of the rest of the work of running our family. Having to leave the house sucks, especially when I really need to be getting to bed and my leaving is likely to escalate the situation. I don't like leaving the sleeping kids there.

Phew-ThatWasClose OP
The couples that make it are the ones that can work together against the common enemy. Almost impossible when half the team is AWOL or worse. Abandonment rage, or RSD, is the second worst sort of extortion. You have to tolerate the verbal abuse otherwise my other disorder will kick in and I'll abuse you even more. Start making an exit plan because PMDD gets worse over time.

Meanwhile, try writing it down. Document everything, of course, so you're ready when the divorce happens. But in the short term try writing down her complaints so they are very clearly heard, acknowledged, and recorded for later discussion. Instead of reacting or greyrocking just write it all down. Interupt the spiral to make sure you have it correct. Ask her to check your work. It ruins the flow and dampens the escalation without being disrespectful. And then there is a clear end. It's all written down, we can go to sleep now.

Check out the forms at IAPMD that I linked to. She may be more willing to create a plan with you than use some template some random yahoo on the Reddit created. The "safety" plan IAPMD put together asks her to identify her triggers. Bring those out into the light so they are specific known things. PMDD makes her cranky and she can "justify" that by claiming a trigger. Well, let's identify those so we can work on avoiding them and lessening their impact.

Ask at Counseling if maybe you could try Rule1. Don't call it that but just say discussing things during luteal hasn't been working so maybe just try not doing that and see if it helps. Also point out in Counseling that taking a timeout is the number one therapist recommended method of dealing with anger. Tell your therapist you heard that somewhere and ask for tips.

Otherwise, if she won't work with you, you're on the countdown. Tolerating abuse is not support. Abuse is never okay. Greyrocking is a survival tactic not a lifestyle. And the kids deserve better.

I wrote this[5], and this (p.117), and this (p.107), and this (p.114).

FarReaction
Thanks. This is very helpful. I am going to try the writing it down

---

5   http://www.reddit.com/r/PMDDpartners/comments/1d49upz

strategy. I will also try bringing the IAPMD forms to counseling.

We have been discussing the "timeout" strategy in counseling and I haven't been able to make any progress. When the PMDD hits, my wife thinks it's stonewalling and neglect if I try to leave, even after sitting there bearing it for a good long while. She says I'm not meeting her emotional needs in those moments; I am finding that I just run out of willpower and discipline to keep holding on in the storm. Usually, it is one of these times that I finally break and leave ("please stop, please just stop, I need a break") that I get my monthly divorce threat ("this time I mean it, I'm calling lawyers.")

> Phew-ThatWasClose OP
> As I mentioned "please stop" was my mantra. I greyrocked for two years because I thought I needed to be there for the kids. But I wasn't actually there. What they really needed was a whole intact person.
>
> Document everything. If she's going to call the lawyers so be it. Take care of yourself.
>
> It's not you. The PMDD has infinite resources. It will push you til you break then call you weak. If you hold on just a little longer … the PMDD will push a little more. Her emotional needs are endless in those moments. An Army of Psychologists couldn't meet her emotional needs.
>
> It's a waste. You end up exhausted and broken and she's not better off. Whatever you do when you can't take it anymore … do that right away. Save your energy, use it for something that makes a difference. Hit the gym, go the coffee shop, whatever.
>
> Counseling should be giving her tools to self sooth. Spinning up berating you is not calming. There's no "getting it out of her system". Turns out it's calming things that help people calm down. Imagine.
>
> I find therapy will just drift if you let it. Go in with an agenda and a goal and most therapists will be happy to help. Let us know how it goes.

Socalwarrior485
Noble. Laudable. Also, completely flawed in my experience.

The moment it starts, all plans go out the window. She goes rogue, nothing is off limits, no rules exist in any way, shape or fashion. Creating rules for partners is what you're proposing, and that's what I have a problem with. If she's under no obligation to follow the rules because she wont, and she's proven that time and again, why should I be held to some standard that she won't hold herself to?

Phew-ThatWasClose OP
Probably won't work the first three, four, five times. But the alternative hasn't worked ... how many times now? It's a plan, not an edict. If the rules go out the window you talk next follicular about why that happened and how that can be fixed. It's iterative. And yes, clearly won't work if there's no buy in.

PMDD gets worse over time so if she won't work with you start planning your exit.

Socalwarrior485
I'm on the back end of it. The buy in faded over time. I'm only pointing out the futility of negotiating with someone who will not uphold their end of the bargain.

Your last point of your comment is right though. If I were 20 years younger, I would have told myself to run. But it didn't show up until after my first child and got significantly worse after the second. My experience with seeing others is that there is no script on how it manifests, nor is there a textbook definition beyond just dysphoria that aligns with menstrual cycles. My wife is effectively disabled without the benefit of a disability support.

Phew-ThatWasClose OP
Peri[6] is a whole other beast. 24/7 and dialed up to 17. Buckle up.

Socalwarrior485
For mine, after the oophorectomy, got way better. Not perfect, but better

theatergeek1
Since 2010 PMDD is listed in the dsm in America as a disability - if you can get the official diagnoses and etc it takes time but maybe you can get disability benefits for her

---

6   http://www.reddit.com/r/PMDD/comments/1f46img/comment/lkow98r

Natural-Honeydew5950
This list is amazing!!!!! I can just change Jane to my own name and it would fit perfectly. I think one thing I would add to is to say, just in case you are not rational right now, write this down and return to it after your period.

> Phew-ThatWasClose OP
> Pretty sure that's in there. Prolly needs to be more prominent.
>
> So bizarre that your SO's name is Simon. :)

Legitimate_Fan8830
My wife eats a bag of Peanut Butter M&Ms during her Doom Week. It's what she requests to cope.

Recently some strangers who discovered this told me I'm a horrible husband and I'm poisoning my wife with sugar. Those people seriously can go f*** themselves.

> GetTheLead_Out
> That's actually hilarious. Sure, a coping mechanism that works for you and her, is cheap, readily available is soooo horrible. /s
>
> Lots of us land on eating less sugar eventually (for blood sugar management, it seems those lows really fuck us to thr stratosphere), but things that work, work.
>
> I drank so many 4 packs of ginger beer for like a year. 1-2 a day (fine, sometimes 3). Haha. If I was out, I needed to stock up.

> Phew-ThatWasClose OP
> I recently discovered there is such a thing as powdered peanut butter. Later that same day I found out protein ice cream is a thing.
>
> It's weird how strangers like to pass judgment.

> > Legitimate_Fan8830
> > Oh yes! I've been hanging out at my friend's house who has a ninja ice cream maker too much lately 😆

IceMalc
I feel you brother. Had the same experience with my ex, who still hasn't owned her PMDD, and says things would have been different if I had been more supportive and understanding!! makes me boil, I was super supportive and understanding but I couldn't help enough, because whatever i did or said was the wrong thing, and she let me know with vitriol. Felt like hurricane was coming when I detected a sudden change of demeanour, and there was nothing I could do to avoid the imminent damage that would occur because never helped her properly with my words and actions. Just became the whipping post.

DontClickTheUpArrow
This all sounds good. Is anyone else's luteal phase a solid 2 weeks? We are pretty match half on and half off. Having to enact this plan 50% of the time just seems so daunting. Also where does sex fall in the plan?

Phew-ThatWasClose OP
It's not going to shorten luteal. Just, hopefully, make it more bearable. And if luteal is more bearable maybe follicular is less about recovery and more about having fun. Then you get into a positive feedback loop and ...

That's the theory anyway. Try it and report back :)

Wtfrank450 - November 29, 2024
You're a legend thanks so much for creating this.

The original post on the sub.[7]

---

7   https://www.reddit.com/r/PMDDpartners/comments/1ftpdv4

From Phew-ThatWasClose

Sample Safety Plan (from the wiki)

If you are not formally diagnosed (p.45) do that. But wait! This can help regardless so read this before you click the link. You have time.

PMDD is a chronic medical condition that affects every member of the family. Like any chronic condition it needs to be managed everyday. During follicular you make a detailed plan *together* for how to navigate the luteal phase. Then everybody knows what to do during luteal. Next follicular you review and revise the plan and improve every cycle.

Mostly the plan during luteal is you pick up extra chores so she can concentrate on self-care. The details are important. Make the plan as concrete, specific, and detailed as possible because luteal is no time to be asking questions. Many women, when they're in the thick of it, can barely talk. So know your job and just get on with it. Check in from time to time, maybe once an hour, but no chit-chat unless she wants to. Even then it's chit-chat only.

Don't forget also to celebrate during follicular. You're together for a reason. Remember why you love each other and recharge those batteries.

Here we have written up what a detailed plan might look like for fictional couple Jane and Simon. We assume Jane has severe PMDD with symptoms like extreme irritability, rage, and despair. We further assume Simon is not an asshole. "Next week" means "when luteal is over". Luteal is generally more like ten days. Whatever.

Sample Safety Plan

0: We will have a period tracking app (e.g.: Stardust[8], Belle[9], Flo[10]) that we both can reference so everybody knows exactly what part of the cycle it is *without having to ask.* (other reminders and signals, if needed, may include: a fire danger spinner on the fridge, marking the paper calendar in the kitchen, a bracelet or sweater Jane wears only during luteal, color coded laminated cards we just leave lying around, etc.)

---

8   http://stardust.app/
9   http://bellehealth.co/
10 http://flo.health/

1: We agree there will be no talking about anything substantive during the luteal phase. This includes finances, major purchases, life goals, regrets, luteal itself, this plan, and The Relationship. If one of us tries to bring up such a topic during luteal the other will say "Let's talk about that next week when we're both in a better place" and that will be a signal or code phrase to drop it for now. Small talk is okay. The local sportsball team or the weather or a silly you saw on the viewscreen.

Certain phrases can also signal the conversation is best left till next week. These include, but are not limited to:

> You always ...
> You never ...
> I just want to say one thing ...
> Can we just talk about this real quick ...
> How come you didn't ...
> I told you to ...
> I probably shouldn't say this but ...
> Can you just listen to me for a second without getting mad ...

If we hear any of these coming out of our own mouth we will immediately stop talking and leave the room. If we hear it coming out of our partners mouth we will say "I love you sweetie. Why don't you write that down and we'll talk about it next week when we're both in a better place."

If for some reason one of the partners is unable to follow Rule 1 the other partner will ask "Can you stop?" If they can they will. If they cannot stop then the partner still able will leave the room. If followed then they will leave the house. If followed they will go for a walk around the neighborhood. The number one doctor recommended way to deal with anger is to <u>take a timeout</u> (p.107).

Each partner will keep a go bag in the car. If it becomes necessary to leave the house for a bit they will go to the gym or the coffee shop or the park or wherever for half an hour to an hour *when it is safe to do so*. Long enough to give the other partner a chance to calm down and interrupt the negative spiral. If it is not safe to use the car, for instance because the other partner is interfering, then both will stay out of the car. The point is to physically separate for a timeout not to just change location. Go for a walk until the other partner goes back inside.

If it's really that important *write it down* so you don't forget. Either partner can do this. We will keep a pad of paper and a pen on the coffee table for just this purpose. Once it's written down we don't have to talk about it anymore. It is heard and acknowledged and recorded. We will discuss it next week.

Once the period of separation is over and both are back in the house, both are calm, Rule 1 still applies and we will not talk about the incident that just happened until next week. At this point it would be good for Simon to make Jane a cup of tea.

2: Managing luteal is difficult and requires everybody's cooperation. Everybody wants to feel safe and cared for. PMDD is a chronic medical condition which makes the luteal phase of Jane's cycle especially difficult both physically and emotionally. To focus on her own health Jane needs Simon to take on most of the household chores. These include:

- Making Dinner: Luteal is not the time to try out that recipe you saw that sounded good. Luteal is a miserable time for Jane and comfort food is paramount. Jane prefers:

  - Boxed mac and cheese because it reminds her of her childhood when she wasn't fucking miserable.
  - Mashed potatoes and gravy - same thing.
  - Burgers (rare because iron is good during luteal)
  - Insert comfort food here.

- Clean the kitchen: Jane has specific ways she likes that done. Simon is not responsible for doing it exactly so. But he will make sure dishes and surfaces are clean and the kitchen is usable for the next meal. The next meal is likely to be Simon making dinner again so it's all good. Any specific bugaboos can be brought up next week.
- Take the trash out: Because it stinks and Jane is especially sensitive to smells during luteal.
- Doing Laundry: Jane likes it done a certain way. Instructions are taped to the wall next to the washer/dryer. Don't do delicates. Jane will take care of that during follicular.

Meanwhile Jane is focusing on self care during Luteal which includes:

- Getting plenty of sleep.
- Drinking plenty of water. (2-3 Liters per day to flush excess cortisol)
- Eating enough, including enough protein, even if junk is all that appeals.
- Not skipping meals and not being hungry because that leads to hangry.
- Taking meds as prescribed and supplements as advised or planned.
- Not supervising Simon as that will just make her upset. He's got this.
- Exercise as able.

- Getting to appointments no matter what.
- Distracting if necessary (Tea, a blanket, and a romcom)
- DBT exercises as needed (rage journaling, powerwalks, heavy bag, puzzles, paper shredding, etc.)

3: Follicular is a good time to try that recipe that looked good. Review and revise the plan to evaluate what worked and what didn't. Make changes as needed, eliminate things that didn't work or didn't serve. Add new stuff to try. Talk about whatever caused the crisis during luteal if there was one. Was there really an issue or just PMDD catastrophizing over something minor?

PMDD is a chronic condition and needs to be managed everyday, even when there are no evident symptoms. This is just the new normal. Anything that promotes general health is going to make luteal easier to manage. Maintain the regimen which means both of us:

- Taking meds as prescribed and supplements as advised or planned.
- Healthy Diet.
- Exercise Daily.
- Getting to appointments and making new ones.
- Research into new and better ways to manage.

Most importantly we will reconnect with each other. Remember how it used to be and do that.

- Socialize with friends.
- Date night
- Netflix & chill
- Individual hobbies
- Together hobbies (that recipe?)

TLDR:

0: Jane will add Simon to her period tracking app as a partner. Simon will download a copy of Jane's period tracking app and *pay attention*.

1: There will be no talking about anything substantive during luteal. If someone really really really wants to because it's so so so important and no honestly this is different and we have have have to talk about it - the other person will leave the house for an hour.

2: Simon will take care of the household during luteal so Jane can focus on self care. Jane will not supervise. Simon will check in every hour or so to see if Jane needs anything. Tea, for example.

3: Reconnect and recharge during Follicular.

The first plan in the collection and in the wiki[11].

---

11 https://www.reddit.com/r/PMDDpartners/wiki/index/bestpractices/samplesafetyplan/

From Specific-Frame8833

Another Safety Plan

Specific-Frame8833 has PMDD.
When asked if she would share her plan[12] this was her response.

Absolutely! Let me first preface this by saying, you have to have a GOOD partner. You truly have to have someone who is good to you. There are a lot of thoughts and feelings that come with PMDD that will make you see your partner in a terrible light. I say this because sometimes I see women talk about their partners that are not good to them 365 days, not just uneducated (in this topic) and unprepared partners during PMDD symptoms. This only works if they have a willingness and openness to understand you and care enough about you to work on ego and pride to support you.

Our plan:

1. Start talking when you're 1 week post period. It's my most mental clarity and it allows me to be more receptive to things I've done/said that were hurtful to my partner and visa versa.

2. Research PMDD together from good sources. Reddit is a great place for anecdotal stories from real women that share similar symptoms. This is great to show to him, not only because it's validating to me, but helps him see that he's probably not alone in the husband world of supporting a wife/partner with PMDD.

3. Kinda bumping back up to 1. Whatever we discuss during that time, we evaluate if we missed a step of the plan to have caused an unwanted interaction or if there's something we need to tweak to not repeat an unwanted interaction.

4. Now for the actual plan. Once I notice symptoms, I vocalize. It usually starts by me being very critical of him. Critical of his facial expressions, tone, the way he closes doors, etc. I notice it based on my reaction to nonverbal communication first. We notice it, we vocalize it, and we start putting the plan in place.

5. From that moment forward, no serious conversations. Anything that requires both of us to have on our thinking caps, we table it. Life happens and if there is something we have to decide on, he writes it down. We have a PMDD journal for this reason. He writes it down and I read it when I'm ready and we don't talk

---

12 https://www.reddit.com/r/PMDDpartners/wiki/index/bestpractices/samplesafetyplan/anotherplan/

about. I respond in the journal. That saves us from arguments and tears every time.

6. We don't really interact. This can seem sad but it works for us. We don't talk in the mornings much at all. He makes breakfast, we eat, and we go on about our days. When he gets home from work, same thing. We may have small talk about our days but don't talk about anything emotionally charged. He will go to the bedroom to read or play video games and I will stay in the living room to read or watch tv. Less interaction just helps. Im annoyed with him and the world. I have less shameful thoughts about wanting to divorce or hating him that cause me to spiral. He has less hurt feelings.

7. He picks up the slack. This might not be for everyone depending on jobs/kids/etc. but my husband has agreed that I don't have to lift a finger. He feeds the cats, he cooks, he cleans, he keeps up with all household chores. If I find the energy to do it, great! If not, it's not an issue. I tend to fall down this spiral during PMDD about how I do all the household chores and start building resentment towards him and it has caused us to have major fights in the past. It's not true, but it's something I started believing every time. So we eliminated that factor completely by taking the task off me during this time.

8. We have PMDD affirmations we use in arguments. If we find ourselves in an argument, my husband has started to just say sorry. Rather than trying to defend himself for something that really, at the end of the day, is nonsensical and not something we'd ever be talking about if it weren't for PMDD, he's gotten really good at just letting it go. (*** this took TWO YEARS. it did NOT happen over night. This step takes WORK and why you have to have a partner willing to let ego and pride go. This isn't an easy task for anyone. Taking the blame for something that is NOT your fault is HARD. If you're reading or trying to implement this step, know that it takes a long time to get here and it's not perfect 100% of the time. We still fight. We still get this wrong. But we've gotten better!) ***Whatever I'm believing in the moment, he's sorry and shows me physical affection (a hug, a kiss, whatever) and then he goes through our affirmations. "You are not a bad person, you are not mean, you are trying to get in control of your body, we love each other, we respect each other, you show kindness, you're a good wife, you're a good friend." It helps center us and we try to get here before it gets out of hand. I'd say we're 80/20 but we're getting better every time.

9. Now this is for the PMDD girlies, it feels REAL. everything you're feeling and thinking feels real. Sometimes it's not. In the same way that my husband says sorry, I do too. When it's over and I hit my shame spiral, I make sure to apologize and let him know his affirmations. He's a good husband, he's a good friend, thank you for being kind, thank you for understanding me, thank you for being 100% when I can only give you 10%. Remind him that he's good and I'm grateful. It will save our relationship.

10. Be kind. I need a lot of affirmations and reassurance during this time. It used to drive my husband wild if I asked are you mad at me and do you love me 60x a day. We've talked and he knows now, just say yes I love you, no I'm not mad. When I'm crying over my lunch because I think he hates me, he doesn't laugh or sigh anymore. He hugs me, rubs my back, and he reassures me. However many times it takes.

11. Probably the most important step for us. Once it's over and we've cleared the PMDD, I plan a date. It helps me feel in control of my body, mind, and emotions and it helps me reconnect with my husband. We try to do 2-3 dates a month. I plan one after PMDD that's all about him. We say it boosts employee morale lol. He plans one for me the next week that's all about me. We plan the 3rd one together to do something we both enjoy.

Overall, the key is to communicate and know when to back down. It's a lot of guessing games and trial and error. We've spent 3 years figuring out what's best for us. This has helped us to get through it without having to go on apology tours for how we acted in the midst of PMDD. my husband is a saint and I couldn't survive this diagnosis without his unwavering support. It's hard but talk about it, write it down, put it into action, and don't quit trying when it fails. Try again. Like I said before, it took us 2 years to get go a place that didn't include wildly out of character behavior on both of our ends during fights. We kept trying. Now we maybe have 1 argument and it's always at the beginning at the start of symptoms. Plans help!

Bonus: go to therapy!! I make sure I always have an appointment scheduled during PMDD/period week and sometimes I use that session just to bitch about my husband. My therapist knows I need it. It's like a filler appointment. It helps me not carry the resentment for a whole week just building to explode.

From 0hh0n3y

I made a notes app on how to help me during PMDD. Use it if it helps!

I sent this through the notes app with my partner. He's a very positive mindset let's just think happy thoughts guy. He also grew up in a natural medicine family and has trouble with medical understanding and why I take meds. I've removed personal details but you can copy and paste or use this as a guide to make your own and add what you want need experience etc. My partner is male and is very much a "how can I fix this" type of guy. So I wanted it to be clear that "you don't!" But here's some ways to HELP:

A Guide to PMDD So we don't both lose our minds.
Snapshot: What is PMDD? PMDD (Premenstrual Dysphoric Disorder) is a severe, hormone-related mood disorder that affects about 5–8% of women. It shows up during the luteal phase (the two weeks before a period) and disappears once menstruation starts. It's not just "bad PMS." It can affect mood, sleep, focus, and relationships.

•   PMDD is not just being cranky or sad before a period •   PMDD is not something I can control with willpower or attitude •   PMDD is not a personality flaw •   PMDD is not fixed by "just being positive"

Why does PMDD happen? PMDD isn't about having too many hormones: it's about the brain overreacting to normal hormone changes. Specifically, my brain is sensitive to estrogen and progesterone shifts, and this sensitivity affects neurotransmitters like serotonin and GABA. Think of it like an allergy: the hormones are normal, but my brain's reaction isn't.

How my medication helps: •   REDACTED

How PMDD affects me personally: Because I know what's happening and manage it with therapy and meds, my symptoms are mild to moderate. Still, stress or sleep disruption can make it worse.

I get: •   Bad insomnia   •   Brain fog   •   Sudden low mood or frustration for no clear reason   •   A sense of "something's wrong" that isn't tied to real events

How do I know I'm in a PMDD cycle? I track it by counting my birth control pills. ● Please don't ask "is this PMS or PMDD?" ☑ Instead: "Hey, want to check where you're at in your pill pack?"

What I need during PMDD: •   Rest   •   Slowness   •   Permission to feel terrible without fixing

I'm not being lazy, dramatic, or unstable. I'm navigating a storm no one else can see. If I'm allowed to go slow and be messy without pressure, I come back faster.

How can you help? DO NOT: •   Cheer me up   •   Tell me it will pass   •   Push me to do more   •   Try to "solve" it with logic or optimism   •   Suggest treatment or "have you tried __"

DO: •   Say "You're okay to feel as sad as you need. I'm still here."   •   Let me move slow   •   Be soft, fuzzy, warm (literally and emotionally)   •   Help me feel like I'm not a burden   •   Ask what would help / treat me like I know what's best for me because I do

"But I'm a guy, I need instructions." Great. Here you go:
☑ Ask about my zone: Example: "Hey just checking in. What color are you today?"   •   Green = Good   •   Yellow = Struggling   •   Red = Barely functioning

☑ Set the vibe: If we're in person: Example: "Let's get you in comfy clothes and I'll make tea."

If we're apart: Example: "I'd order you sushi and let you lay on the couch watching something dumb. Since I can't, let's pick a dumb show to watch together."

☑ Make me feel safe: Say: "I know this isn't forever. I'm not going anywhere. I'm here. Let's just finish today together."
Don't push me to be "better" tomorrow. That adds pressure even if well intended.

☑ Ask calmly if I need space: "Hey, I want to be here for you. But I also get the sense you might need some solo time. Want me to check back in an hour?"

☑ If you're physically here: •   Get sushi. Get snacks. Get the good food!   •   Write a dumb sticky note   •   Refill my water   •   Put on a stupid movie   •   Do one small thing I'll pick up on it   •   Help me with 1 chore

One last thing: You don't have to understand PMDD to be great at helping me through it. You just have to meet me where I am. The storm always passes but I remember who helped me feel safe during it. 💜

The original comment on the sub.[13]

---

13 https://www.reddit.com/r/PMDD/comments/1k6n0mh

From SophiaFalconePMDD

Here's our Plan... it's silly and short.

Clair = me with the PMDD
Torval = my awesome partner

1. Safety first. Includes driving while angry for both Clair and Torval. Torval do your best not to engage and leave the scene for your own well-being. Clair will be fine.

2. Torval - You are a great and loving partner. Remember.

3. Torval, if you engage Clair, oops – it doesn't matter! Nothing to be disappointed over, it happens when you are being attacked. Move on, see #2.

4. Clair is not to text Torval during luteal. Only appropriate texts are "On my way" and "I love you" or combo of there of ?

5. Torval is not to answer texts that spill through when rule #4 is violated by Clair.

6. Torval is to remember that Clair can not communicate well verbally when her brain is overwhelmed. Assume answers are not intended to be short, and that non-answers = slow processing of data, not intentional ignorance.

7. If Clair moves way quickly and abruptly to another room or out of the house without communicating it was because quick action was needed and it's no reflection on Torval. See #2.

8. If Clair needs to go to parents or out, also not a reflection on Torval and the support he provides.

This one is in <u>the wiki</u>[14].

---

14 https://www.reddit.com/r/PMDDpartners/wiki/index/bestpractices/samplesafetyplan/falcone/

From Agitated_Ad9471

donivan-floyd - April 30, 2025

Love my girl, just need some encouragement!

Howdy! My Fiance and I have been together around 2 years, and actively learning a lot about her PMDD! I would like to preface that Her and I have a tremendous relationship, and I am proud of what we have worked through! I suppose this time around, in the heat of PMDD... I feel I am losing track of some of the basics! Does anybody else get caught off guard and feel like they are scrambling for the right approach to help her (or maybe leave her alone if that's what's helping)? I am looking for maybe some wisdom about how to stay grounded, and serve with a good intention. I feel like the selfish desires really push on me, and I choose to forget that she is really struggling. I do not want to put up my guard, and I desire to act with compassion and patience! Any uplifting thoughts, stories? I love the heck out of her, and I am dedicated to process... just maybe looking for some tools to add to my tool belt! Thanks!

Agitated_Ad9471
Tracking her cycle is really beneficial to her and you. It gives perspective on things and helps you to prepare. My boyfriend and I are almost at 4yrs together and we're always learning new things and growing together to help our relationship/ PMDD. I feel like the more we learn, grow and both work together the easier handling PMDD has become and our overall relationship. We have protocols and safewords in place and prioritise communicating how we're feeling. best relationship we've both been in. So much love and respect for each other because we both put in the work

donivan-floyd OP
Fantastic, thank you! Could you give me an example of what a safe word / protocol may look like... so I may think of a personal situation it may be useful in? Thanks again!

Agitated_Ad9471
Yeah for sure. Protocols like not talking about problems in luteal, saving heavy stuff for follicular. Try not to make big plans in luteal and work around that time, as we're feeling physically and mentally depleted. Making sure to have meds/ supplements and remedies - evening primrose, premular, b6, iron ect. Rescue remedy (drops or

chews). As there's a link to a serotonin deficiency in pmdd, doing something to increase that (eg, dancing, walking, swimming ect) during luteal is paramount. Also making sure I sleep and eat enough in luteal has been a big one for me. pmdd makes you get insomnia real bad so when I'm in ovulation I'll sleep very little and in luteal I'll sleep a lot, often needing naps. My bf is really understanding of this and helps me prioritise sleep. I also struggle to feed myself during luteal and that usually makes things a lot worse, the hanger is real 😵 my bf helping with getting good food organised is a godsend, it helps immensely and it's something I really appreciate of him 🥺

In terms of safewords - when I'm overstimulated and need to be left alone to recharge and collect myself, I'll tell bf im going to go unwind - he knows that means I love him but need space, I'll be outside having a gummy, unwinding and I'll be in when I'm in a better space. Sometimes I can communicate this but sometimes my mouth and brain don't work/connect and just saying a safeword is helpful.

Another thing we've learnt is calling my pmdd thoughts/feelings a name so it feels separate, after all it does feel like someone else has taken over my body/thoughts during that time. I use the name Regina (after Regina George lol) cause it does feel like I'm being bullied by a cruel teenager. When I get fucked up pmdd thoughts I'll say 'shut the fuck up Regina, you don't know what you're on about' and it helps lol. It's also a way to tell my bf pmdd is kicking my ass. 'Regina is being a right bitch to me again' and he'll say back 'stop being mean to my gf Regina!', it's cute.

Hope that makes sense, I'm dyslexic and ready for a nap lol

donivan-floyd OP
Thank you so much, definitely some really good strategies here! I am also thankful that you were so detailed in your response, I really appreciate you taking the time to write it! I am excited to look more into those vitamins, and maybe helping my lady meal prep… that's huge! I will take this to heart!

The original post at the sub.[15]

---

15 https://www.reddit.com/r/PMDDpartners/comments/1kc09y1

From Remarkable-Banana512

I am in a LTR / cohabitate with an absolute saint of a man. I believe the two most difficult things for him are:

1. Feeling like I'm trying to hold him accountable for things that are not his fault (my feelings are big, he didn't "let me" get enough rest, he said something harmless that i took personally, I'm mean to him but expect him to be extra sweet to me, he didn't get the very specific food that is the only thing that sounds appetizing to me, etc)

2. Feeling helpless and having to watch me suffer every single month

I can't speak for him, but some things I've seen work for us: Issue 1:

- i have a period tracker and keep him informed of where i am in my cycle. this helps him be sensitive to me and it helps me know where im at

- i encourage (but try not to push) him to make plans with his friends and coworkers and to go out for his own activities (running, watching a game at a bar, easy things he likes to do by himself anyway) so he gets some "fresh air" while I burrow and sulk. When he comes home I try to ask him about it :) it's easy conversation for me because I just get to go "tell me more" and he gets to tell me about his day

- we do very easy, low stakes things with each other: go out to a see a movie or watch one inside, paint together, do a puzzle, make a pizza. Things that don't require a lot of energy and that can be put down very easily if i get frustrated or overwhelmed

- for me, it's difficult but i try to be very aware of when my feelings are not lining up with my reality. I know we have a very loving relationship but on my period i think things like "he doesn't understand" or "he just wants to push me to do everything like normal" or "he's going to get sick of me. he hates me when i act like this." I journal these feelings and then rip up the pages so i can express the frustration without building a catalog of hate. I also TRY to balance this by journaling about the positive, especially when im off my period and am thinking more clearly. This helps me keep the positive/truthful things in mind when I am feeling bonkers.

- AFTER MY CYCLE WHEN I AM TRULY RECOVERED I ask him if I said or did anything on my period that still affects or hurts him and I apologize. It's very important this happens after my cycle so i can actually hear him and be rational. Again, I can't speak for him but I think this helps him know that I really do care about him and don't expect him to just put up with 7+ days of me being a wreck without any acknowledgement of what he goes through as my partner. I also do my best to reflect on how he supported me and thank him for those specific things.

- my partner loves physical touch, especially a good back/foot rub, and that's a very easy way for me to show him my appreciation. Maybe there's something your partner enjoys that you can do special for him?

Issue 2:

- he makes me a steak or red meat of some sort on my first day of bleeding. Not only does the extra iron help me (and generally makes me feel very spoiled to have a special meal just for me, the man doesn't even eat meat) but I know he likes to feel like he's able to help me in a tangible way

- he brings me water, draws a bath, gets me snacks (I crave chocolate and hot Cheeto fries usually). Again this does double duty of helping me feel very cared for and he feels like he's able to help me. It's also very easy to express gratitude for delicious snacks.

The other thing that helps me, take it or leave it (as with all advice) is weed. I can go from completely overwhelmed to the point of just wanting to die to pretty chill gal in a matter of 2-3 hits if a joint. CBD joints aren't as effective but they help too when I need to calm down but don't want to be stoned. Idk if you guys smoke / if it's legal where you are, but we do "stoney walks" and have cozy nights very frequently when I'm on my period. It elevates my mood like no SSRI can.

Oh and I've also mastered the phrase "my crazy brain is telling me xyz…im sorry in advance if im sensitive or snappy today". It's not a blank check to act however I feel in the moment but it helps us both be on the same page about what's going on. I also use DBT skills to help ground myself if I start feeling very extreme.

It's very difficult to be a person with PMDD and I know it's difficult for our partners too. I encourage you to have a lot of empathy and compassion for yourself and to try to remember (especially on your period) that this is something that is happening TO you and that you are a TEAM against this ugly monster that comes in and ruins our mental and physical health every month.

Sorry to have written an essay, I hope at least some of this is helpful!

The original comment in a now deleted post.[16]

---

16 https://www.reddit.com/r/PMDD/comments/1m0ql6x/comment/n3bl59o

It's time for YOU (us) to take some responsibility

(Editors note: Included the whole post and 36 comments. People kept finding it and discussion lasted almost two years. Well worth reading the whole thing.)

Dontwakethellama - March 4, 2024

Hey there. We're in the PMDD Partners sub and it's a safe space to vent and seek advice for some of the trickier situations that we find ourselves in.

However, I see countless posts echoing the same frustration – partners feeling defeated, taking the blame, and enduring mental/verbal abuse during their partner's PMDD luteal phase.

Look, I get it. You care deeply and want to support your partner, but being a doormat isn't the answer.

Coming from my experience:

Stop enabling the unhealthy behavior... Take responsibility for the next steps and lead your partner through each phase. Absorbing blame, apologizing for non-existent faults, and accepting abuse are not acts of love; they're enabling the PMDD symptoms to control the relationship.

It's crucial to remember two things:

PMDD is real, and **it's not an excuse for abuse**. When (not if) they can't control themselves, it's up to you to take control by disengaging. It's like arguing politics with someone who doesn't believe the same things as you... You're NEVER going to convince them, no matter how solid your facts are. Walk away.

You are not powerless. You have the right to set boundaries and prioritize your own well-being.

Here's a different approach that helped me and my partner:

Educate yourselves: Together, research PMDD and explore resources to understand the condition better. Knowledge empowers you both to navigate challenges. The way I have explained it to people is "bipolar disorder on a monthly schedule".

Communicate openly, and firmly: Express your needs and concerns clearly, and don't accept blame for their actions. You'll see me repeat this multiple times - communication needs to happen mostly during her "normal" time. Once the luteal phase kicks in, your communication mostly becomes disengagement.

Establish boundaries (and stick to them): Decide what behaviors you will not tolerate, and calmly but firmly disengage when those lines are crossed. This isn't about punishment; it's about protecting yourself. It helps her as well... How many times have you heard the apologizing and shame after she comes out of it? If you disengage, you may save her from saying/doing something that shes ashamed about later. I said this in a previous post, and it struck a chord with a few people, so I'll repeat it here: Create the boundaries together when you're both in a good state of mind, then honor your promises to THAT version of your partner. She will be back, and she's counting on you.

Track the cycles TOGETHER: Don't leave it up to her, and don't secretly do it and pull it out of your back pocket as a "gotcha" when she starts acting differently. Also, bring it up! Set a calendar invite for a few days prior to when you know it's going to start and acknowledge that it's coming, together. Then, when it starts, remind her that you love her and that you can tell that she's starting to not feel great and that you are going to follow the boundary protocol that you both established prior (going for a walk, sleeping in the other room, calling a friend, etc).

Don't use it as a tool to shut her down, and also don't be afraid to say it out of fear of making her upset. If you've both prepped for this, then it's not the same as the old blaming the period trope. It's an acknowledgement of it to bring both of your awarenesses to it.

Focus on solutions, not blame games: When things get tense, it's ok to still try to find solutions that work for both of you. You MAY be able to have discussions like "what would make this better for you right now?". If the answer is "I wish you/I were dead" or something not productive, then disengage... but if it's "I just wish you would stop talking", then BOOM! You know exactly what (not) to do.

Seek professional help: No matter your financial situation, you *need* to seek therapists and doctors experienced in PMDD (it's actually pretty hard to find, but they're out there). Ultimately, we found that no medications actually work to *cure* it... But medication induced menopause has changed the game for us. It's almost like she doesn't have PMDD at all... She's happy, energetic, motivated, and has her sex drive back! We're about halfway through a 3 month trial. If it continues, then we will go for surgical menopause to make it permanent.

It won't be easy, but by taking charge of your well-being, communicating openly, and setting healthy boundaries, you can create a more balanced and supportive environment in your relationship. Remember, you deserve to be treated with respect, and you're not alone.

I'd like this to be a discussion. Ask questions and contribute your experience with what worked and what didn't work. If you get advice and think "I don't think that would work in my specific situation" get over that for a second and try it with an open mind (if you go into it thinking it will fail, then it will). I -would- like to limit the "if you aren't married or have kids, then get out now" advice. It might be a solution, and it isn't the only solution... If someone is seeking advice, they're interested finding ways to make it work because someone they love is suffering.

**** This is directed more at the PMDD sufferers that lurk here... Not an attack from me, I just want to make an appeal to you ****

Some people get all "no chemicals in my body" in response to me suggesting chemical menopause... But, literally think of the alternative. Let's say you're in your thirties, you have 20ish more years of this... Every... Month. Is it not worth potentially stopping this? If we can agree that this is miserable every month, then you're saying that knowing you're going to live miserably for 20 years is worth it? There's a chance you could live happily, but you don't want to? That's just a bit absurd to me. Or another viewpoint: You've been planning to have kids and don't want to give that option up... But, do you really want to have a child dealing with a mother that is hot/cold every month? It will be confusing. You won't mean to do it, but you'll be mentally/emotionally abusive to these kids. You have to set aside your preconceived ideas of what you want to do and really look at the reality of your situation. Life isn't fair, and you need to make choices that reflect the actual position you're in. Someone who goes blind doesn't get to drive racecars or fly planes like they wanted to their whole life... You have to work with the hand you're dealt.

HusbandofPMDD
Thank you for the thoughtfulness and care that you put into this. Lots of good things to think about.

I get that some partners resist any kind of medicine, but even with OTC meds a significant improvement can be acheived. Life can be so much better with medicine, therapy, accountability, and both people working together.

Greenleaf45678

What kinds of medicine?

> HusbandofPMDD Are you asking what potential solutions are?
> There is chemical menopause (that OP refers to). This is generally
> short-term and simulates what would happen after menopause or an
> oophorectomy.
>
> There is also birth control (some people find that this helps,
> depending on the type of BC)
>
> There are SSRIs (taken either during luteal phase (uniquely effective
> in PMDD sufferers), or throughout the cycle) - this can cause a
> significant improvement.
>
> There are OTC supplements (there's a huge range here, with again
> mixed effectiveness, from 5-htp, to Dim, to Vitex, to ashwagandha,
> and anti-histamines, often used in combination, sometimes for the
> whole cycle, some just for luteal phase).
>
> There are probably more.

Phew-ThatWasClose
That is awesome Llama! Thanks for doing that. We should make it sticky
or something.

Time-Place5719
Impressive post! Personally, I've been navigating this for more than three
years – a potential divorce, and my wife entrenched in denial. The
catalyst? It all began when she directed her focus towards my daughter.
Armed with my knowledge of her triggers, she zeroed in on the kids.
PMDD/PME is unquestionably real, and so is the denial. I firmly believing
she's experiencing bipolar disorder traits – a "bipolar disorder on a
monthly schedule!" Everything aligns with my experience! I'd also
incorporate attachment styles and trauma bonding as products of PMDD.

> dontwakethellama OP
> Your last part about attachment styles and trauma bonding is
> something that I've been trying to learn more about. It seems incredibly
> common that people with PMDD have anxious or fearful attachment
> styles in relationships.

Living in fear or having extreme anxiety around attachment from early in life would definitely have an effect on hormonal response and cortisol levels. I wonder if there have been any studies that show how the body's heightened chemical response affects those individuals as adults.

My understanding is that it's not a direct increase or decrease of hormone levels that causes extreme behavior changes, but the fluctuation itself, which could be up or down or variable. The treatment that my wife is receiving has stopped the estrogen production in her body, which was unstable and not consistent. Now, she wears a patch that has a constant and steady supply of estrogen and progesterone… The steady release is what we're being told is what makes the difference. All signs are pointing to that being accurate.

> Time-Place5719
> Trauma bonding takes hold when you find yourself consistently trying to please your wife or apologizing for various things (unfounded accusations). The dynamic becomes so unhealthy that it literally creates a trauma bond (our professional confirmed we have experienced the attachment styles). You start questioning whether you're a good person, husband, professional, etc., and it feels like you're constantly walking on eggshells. Stonewalling, criticism, contempt, defensiveness – that's the cycle created by a hormonal imbalance that affects maybe the way reality is perceived: Rejections Sensitivity Dysphoria! Please see this: I came across a doctoral thesis discussing attachment styles and PMDD. https://digitalcommons.liberty.edu/cgi/viewcontent.cgi?article=5902&context=doctoral[17]

zumafan
This is only helpful to those who have partners that acknowledge they have a problem/condition. If you have a partner that refuses to believe they have a problem, and everything is your fault, none of these things will work. Just sayin.

> Temporary-County-356
> Which is what he is saying, you don't need to be doormat. You deserve peace and respect every single day. I don't care what anyone else's say. You need to advocate for yourself. Life is way too short. To be dealing with things that aren't bringing you joy. Most suffering is what

---

17 http://digitalcommons.liberty.edu/cgi/viewcontent.cgi?article=5902&context=doctoral

people put up with from other people. Take these people out of your life and boom peace of mind. I believe a lot of people are co-dependent and don't like change. So the devil they know is better than one unknown or being by themselves. Which is bizarre. Don't be a doormat.

Time-Place5719
Absolutely! I maintained a balance for three years, but it's not sustainable. Sooner or later, everything is bound to implode.

> dontwakethellama OP
> It could, and I don't think everything is predestined any certain way. There are always conversations that can be had to help open their mind… Maybe their partner is not the right person to have that conversation. Someone else outside the relationship may have a bigger impact on getting someone to recognize that there's an issue
>
> I mentioned in another post that I had resigned myself to a semi-fulfilled life. That was while I was having all of these conversations and plans etc. It was exhausting and I felt like I got a partial relationship. That's why I say you have to get her professional care.
>
> Her not going because of pride or money or whatever is what you have to look at. If she admits there's an issue and is unwilling to do anything about it, that's where you have to get serious.… Like an alcoholic that doesn't admit they have a problem.
>
> My perspective is definitely one with a partner that admits and acknowledges the issue at hand, and I value the alternate viewpoints as well! It's all helpful for the sub!

> > Time-Place5719
> > I'm currently navigating through this process. I've laid out everything for our psychologist – even shared details about this forum, Videos, academic articles, conferences about partners, etc… I genuinely believe I'm taking the right steps, perhaps my final attempt. Specifically, I'm confident that our psychologist believes me, and in the initial sessions, she's addressing emotional dysregulation. Handling the denial is delicate; it needs a cautious approach to prevent her from avoiding sessions. I hope the therapist is patiently waiting for the opportune moment to broach the topic – that's my last hope.

Efficient-Pattern189
That part right there !!

Phew-ThatWasClose
Walking away is always an option. If she's going to spiral anyway let her do it without you.

dontwakethellama OP
Hey Zumafan, I agree with you that your partner does need to be self-aware enough to recognize a cyclical issue. Even if it's just that your relationship struggles every month for part of it and then is great for the other part.

That requires a conversation with her to let her know what the experience is like for you and that you want to put up boundaries on what you will accept in your relationship.

For example, when she's feeling better: "Hey Ms Zumafan, can we talk about the arguments we had last week? When you said ______ and ______, I felt really hurt. I was trying to (Make your night great by taking care of chores — make dinner — enjoy a conversation with my friend) and it seemed like your anger was directed at me... Was there something else going on? Can you explain what it is that I did that made you upset?"

In my experience, my wife concedes that it wasn't me and she was just having a bad day... She apologizes... Then the conversation continues.
"So, have you noticed that this seems to happen every month around the same time? Can we start looking out for that to see if it has a pattern? Also, in the future, if our arguments start getting too heated for either of us, I'd like us to agree that either one of us can request to pause the argument and come back to the disagreement later when we've both cooled down. I don't want either of us to get so mad that we hurt each other's feelings"

She will likely agree because she's thinking rationally and that sounds like a healthy relationship thing to do.

Now, when it comes up again and you're in the heat of it all, you have to start getting REALLY GOOD at recognizing that it's not just a normal argument. Defending yourself won't work and there is nothing to prove. It's time to say "hey, I think that I'd like to pause this like we discussed and we can talk about it later." THEN STICK TO IT! Don't get pulled back into the boiling pot of water. Step away and do whatever it is you planned WITH HER when she was herself.

If that doesn't work, then you get to edit the plan and try something else next week. This goes back to my point of TAKE RESPONSIBILITY.
Again, keep her in the loop. "Last week, when we were arguing, I went to the guest room but then you came in the room and wanted to continue the argument. So, I request that you stick to our plan AND, if we start arguing again, I'm going to go for a drive/walk/hike/etc so we can BOTH have some peace. I'm not leaving you, I'm just letting us calm down and then I'll be back" (that line helped with my wife's fear of abandonment)

These are things that worked for me. Put your own special flavor on it, but keep the structure and framing of it the same. You aren't doing these things for YOU, you're doing it for US. It isn't just YOU that has the option to step away, it's her too… Come at the conversation in a way that is collaborative so she has a say and can offer input while you're also setting yourself up for agreed upon ways to deescalate. The hope is that she'll remember your conversation in that moment and will accept it because she also was a part of that decision/plan. She may give attitude and say "ok, whatever… Walk away", and that's ok. Don't reengage with that. The plan worked… You are now walking away instead of continuing that argument.

dontwakethellama OP
Also, my perspective is definitely one with a partner that admits and acknowledges the issue at hand, and I value the alternate viewpoints as well! It's all helpful for the sub!

Time-Place5719
She told me last night, "Nobody asked you to be my caregiver!" I get it, it's the luteal phase, with dark eyes and a cloud of depression. I'm still compassionate. But the denial takes it to another level – confabulating with friends and parents, all to defend the notion that women can't be abusive, and it's always the man's role!

dontwakethellama OP

The compassion that you have for your wife... Do you have that for yourself?

The narrative around abuse... Yeah... As a man myself, I know what you mean. It's just another thing to navigate. Don't let it stop you. Have some tact though... Don't go and tell everyone that she's abusive unless they have the power to stop it or to help you. If they're just an ear for you to vent that to, then you're gossiping.

> Time-Place5719
> Certainly! However, the nature of abuse in this scenario is unique. It's remarkable to think about how the dynamics influenced by attachment styles can obscure the genuine intent behind the abuse. In my view, the core objective of this abuse is to avoid personal pain and, instead, to project or impose that inner pain onto another person. These dynamics may give rise to tangible manifestations such as criticism, stonewalling, contentp, and a sense of defenselessness. Even though it's linked to PMDD, the experience feels undeniably real and is internalized as such by PMDD sufferers. Nobody can see it...
>
> Ironically, in certain cases, including my own, the abuser has turned into the victim.

Efficient-Pattern189
The denial

Justchristinen
PMDD sufferer here, married for 10 years. I'm 40. I'm doing the chemical menopause (Orilissa is the medication) and it's been amazing. I've been suffering with this since I was 12 and have tried everything under the sun. You can stop at anytime and I haven't noticed any side effects. Certainly less than SSRIs.

> dontwakethellama OP
> I'm really glad that you have found relief, and thank you for sharing! Some quick questions if you're open: How long have you been taking Orilissa? What are the reasons that you would stop? When you stopped, did the PMDD Simpsons kick back in?
>
> > Justchristinen

> I'm so sorry I just saw this! I've been on orilissa for over a year now. I would only stop if there was a detriment to my health, but I just had bone density and other tests and all is good. I got really sick in the fall and couldn't take my meds for about a month and oh boy did it kick in again.
>
> I think the plan is to stay on this for a few years and then maybe address surgery, still not sure!

Time-Place5719
This interview is so revealing: https://youtu.be/kXYw3o9sROA?si=276x1WDuhO1pDpcV[18]

chilllpill
I agree with this advice, but it's hard when the verbal assaults turn physical when you stonewall, disengage, or walk away, as this makes my partner feel blamed or that I am "holier than though" (even if I am sure not to abandon her and will caveat with "I love you and going to take a 5 minute walk to clear my head and come back to resume).

I also wonder what you make of the partner saying "so based on the fact that you ___, would you agree you've been abusive to me?" And if I say anything but "yes" it leads to a massive explosive reaction. Is admitting "fault" when there is none, simply to avoid further conflict, the same as being a doormat?

And then on top of it my partner saying "And this is NOT PMDD talking, this is me and how I really feel because I feel this way the rest of the month too." Do I trust that, or anything she says, during PMDD?

> dontwakethellama OP
> I feel you on this stuff, and I immediately want to address your first topic: Physical abuse shall not be tolerated. You wouldn't get a free pass to come home drunk (out of your normal state of mind) and slap her (nor should you).
>
> I will also reiterate that a lot of the WORK is done between cycles. You talk with her while she's in her good mood... No relationship is perfect, so that means you have to create a safe space to actually air out all the dirty laundry that is real. If she says "I feel like you care more about

---

18 https://youtu.be/kXYw3o9sROA?si=276x1WDuhO1pDpcV

_____ than our relationship" or "it sucks when you __", that is a time for you to accept that responsibility, don't defend… You're only defending against how she feels and telling her she's wrong is invalidating those feelings. Instead, say something like "I didn't know that when I do __ that it makes you feel that way." Then, come up with a way that you can alleviate that issue… Or ask her. It's better if you at least try to come up with a solution and ask if it would help instead of putting all the work on her. If your solution isn't received well, THEN ask if she has a better solution in mind. If you agree to it, then follow through… No lip service please. Set a calendar reminder for yourself if it's something like housework… Figure out a way to solve what you KNOW could cause it to fall apart.

This will be ongoing… It should be in every relationship, so learn it now and repeat it forever.

So let's get back to PMDD stuff… All the work you do between cycles is practice, and the Luteal phase is the big game. You have come up with agreements for how to handle things if they go sideways… If that is to stonewall, disengage, or walk away, then you do that. I would not suggest stonewalling or disengaging without verbally acknowledging it though. A simple "hey, this is getting too intense and I'd like for us to talk about this later. I'm going to go for a walk like we talked about".

So now, you find that you lost the game… Things didn't go well. Ok, what went wrong? What went right? Make adjustments and have conversations.

Do not believe anything she says during the luteal phase when it comes to lashing out at you. She may say she feels that way all the time, but you just talked to her when she was clear headed and she said that wasn't an issue. She is fully coherent and aware, but her reality has shifted… She may believe 100% that she feels this way all the time, but that may not be the case.

It also could be the case, and you just need to make sure that your conversations during practice are open and safe. She should feel safe to admit something to you that could make you angry, and you need to NOT react with anger or abandonment. Ask questions… Get curious… Get a clear understanding… Then acknowledge "I can see how that could feel that way". Then you either apologize and offer a solution or share the part of the story that she may not know as to why you're acting that way.

A lot of the conversations I'm talking about may be better with a professional present… Write down a list of things that you're going to talk about before you go. They will likely ask "what do we want to discuss today" and then you have a guide for what you're going to work through. If the list is long, bring up the topics that you think have the most chance of going haywire so the professional can reel you both back… Or maybe even help dig deeper into the root causes of the feelings.

What are your thoughts on all of this? I know I dropped a lot on ya.

Phew-ThatWasClose
This all needs to stop. Physical abuse is not okay, but neither is verbal abuse. And declaring that walking away is equivalent to an acusation is textbook victim blaming. The RVO in DARVO. That is coercive and manipulative in an effort to get you to stay and endure more abuse.

Forced confessions and apologies naturally follow. 'Either agree with me or I will explode' is just raw intimidation. In some places that is legally defined as abuse. You're not a doormat. You're doing what you need to do to survive. The mistake is being there.

"This is not PMDD" screamed in rage during the Luteal phase absolutely is PMDD. And likely something else thrown in. As Llama points out the game is lost at that point. Just get through this luteal phase with minimal damage, regroup, and figure it out during the next follicular.

The best way to get through a highly charged luteal phase with minimal damage is to leave. If she tries to pull you back in with the "hollier than thou" BS leave faster and further. Tell her you'll be back, but not to resume. You'll talk next week.

Tolerating abuse is not support. And tolerating More abuse because she's blame shifting validates the nonsense at great cost to you. You need those resources to do the work when it counts. Next week during follicular.

Don't spend time and energy being the target of her rage. It helps no one. You get trashed and she spirals out of control. Now she has rage And regret. Without you there the rage sputters and fades. Lashing out at the air. Still not good, but less bad.

Stay safe.

chilllpill
I appreciate hearing all of this. The only wrench in the "leave for a week and regroup" plan is our small child. I can't leave him with her (she says she doesn't have the ability to care for him alone), I can't take him with me (she won't allow it, probably fearing I won't bring him back). So it's me sticking it out while enduring all kinds of abuse along the way.

Phew-ThatWasClose
Yeah, it's hard with kids involved. All the more reason to get this relationship back on track. That kid deserves better.

I didn't say leave for a week. Just leave for an hour, a half hour, ten minutes. Something to disrupt the verbal abuse, catch a breath, and recover your balance.

Go get a pint of ice cream, bring it home, and talk about anything else. Politics. How about that SOTU? Or nothing else. Eat ice cream in silence. Practice intentionality.

Verbal abuse is not acceptable ever, definitely not with the kid there. Nothing can be accomplished during luteal. Stop arguing. Talk about it "next week" once the luteal phase is over. If there is a legitimate concern you can address it when everybody is calmer.

And that's now? It's been almost a week. Has she started her period? Go read the wiki. Specifically the part about creating a safety plan.

She recognizes she's not fabulous during that part of her cycle. The kid needs two functioning parents. "What can WE do to make OUR kids home a warm loving environment to grow up in?"

The low hanging fruit is getting the PMDD under control. Vitamins? Supplements? BC? SSRI? Now is the time to make doctors appointments, do more research, stock the freezer, and make a plan.

This cycle went badly. Neither one of you wants to repeat next cycle. Commit now to not arguing next luteal. And figure out how to shut it down when it starts. It'll be hard, but better with practice.

Reach out if you want to chat.

Workaccount1138 – February 25, 2025
Bruh - I grew up with my dad fitting the role you enjoy with your wife and child.

I found my way into repeating the cycle now with my wife after growing up within that flavor of wildly dysfunctional household emotional snd interpersonal relationship fucked up dynamics—which had historically consisted largely of a matriarch who has extremely immature emotional development and emotional handling capabilities,

…as well as near-zero self awareness of what kind of harm is being done to those people unfortunate enough to be in close proximity to any radically-self-unaware matriarch who compulsively and consistently introduces unfettered, unnecessary, illogical chaos into one's home life.

unless you want this shit to become a lifelong afflicting, continuously-reoccurring, insurmountable, quality of life reducing repeated illnesses and lifestyle hurdle….for your child(s) as they grow into adulthood…

you need to do two things:

1. quietly and PRIVATELY begin building a massive paper trail about your partner's dysfunctional tendencies—as well as any mitigating efforts and strategies and actions you have taken and continue to pursue in your life and in care + love for your family—including your partner and children;

2. force an ultimatum but ONLY AFTER you have first allocated considerably-adequate time and effort while building enough paper trail to take custody of your child by force if things go south.

you owe the children stability and safety above all else. you do this by ensuring that their physical custody is secure and cannot be taken from you by an unwell partner/mom and wife, nor any biased or hostile or lazy family courts system in a child custody/marital separation context.

3. you force your wife's hand into REAL MEANINGFUL personal and mental wellness structured development and healing activities. professional medical service providers with regimented,

structured, formal treatment plans that MUST be adhered to diligently and compliantly by your partner for your relationship to continue existing.

Any continued failure or unwillingness to abide by the terms of this arrangement and understanding will absolutely lead to and can be assumed to result in a separation of you & your partner, in addition to the dissolution of the marriage between you and your partner.

you owe your kid(s) stability, as does your wife. you cannot force your wife's hand into doing anything she does not want or that she refused accept must be done. you can only encourage and if necessary, separate yourself and your children and remove you and yours from the crazy chaotic equation your wife is single handedly introducing into you and yours children's home and lives.

put your foot down for your kids my man.

doblador_de_tierra November 23, 2024
I really appreciate the care, attention, and empathy you put into this post (kind of up until that last part and I'll explain why). I have recently started to suspect I have PMDD after years of dealing with anxiety and depression that only got worse the weeks leading up to my period. I also have ADHD which is an additional layer of complication. My partner is an angel and my rock, and both of our respective mental health struggles have only helped us learn how to communicate better with each other, and in turn with those we love around us. It took a lot of self awareness, reflection, and ultimately accountability to make this 6 year relationship work. I have always struggled with loving myself, and that was truly the first step I needed to take in order to take action. I needed to care deeply about myself, I thought I cared but I didn't. Letting this monster that is PMDD go on to ruin my life was not caring and loving myself, not getting help even though I knew I needed it was absolutely not an act of self love — I think people that turn themselves into victims in these scenarios THINK they are watching out for themselves, but they are not, they are making excuses for behaviors I KNOW they hate because I really grew to hate the person I was leading up to my period. I love my boyfriend, and I want to treat him with love and respect, but am I even taking the time to love and respect myself first? I wasn't. That's when I took action. I am now happily medicated, it saved my life, and it is saving my relationship.

I think what I struggle with (as I said I'm medicated) with your last paragraph, is the switch up in empathy when you decided to address the PMDD lurkers. Our healthcare system has always prioritized the health and safety of men, and there is so much we don't know about women's health because we are not being represented, heard or prioritized. I always say that if a man has to live as a woman for a year, they would NOT be able to handle the degradation, invisibleness, and assumed ignorance we have to walk around with constantly. It is frustrating and infuriating and traumatizing to live in a world that is structurally not built for us. I agree with you that it is tough seeing someone you know needs help, you know their life could improve if they just took the time to at least TRY medication or therapy. But telling the lurkers who are struggling with this form of self love that they are absurd and should consider not having children is not going to do anything to open up the productive conversation we actually need to have for these PMDD sufferers to take the first step to relieve their symptoms.

dontwakethellama OP
Hi, I'm glad you were able to get some value from what I wrote. PMDD is something that I repeatedly say I would never wish upon my worst enemy, let alone people I love and care about. It is always good to hear that people are able to get the symptoms under control and are able to see things from a neutral perspective instead of taking on the role of a victim or even embracing the opposite aggressor role.

I'm sorry that my ending was a bit abrupt and, admittedly, confrontational. My reason for ending that way was because I had seen multiple posts from partners in this sub that were venting. They were upset and hurt by their own partner and needed a safe place to let out their emotions and to seek support, only to be attacked in the comments by PMDD sufferers telling them that their feelings of hurt are invalid for whatever reason. I wanted to cut that off at the head. I wanted to make a post that was tough love for the partners... I have a feeling that my post telling the members of this sub to take responsibility was a bit confrontational and required reading with an open mind. Attacks and invalidation in the comments could have put up defensiveness at my attempted appeal.

I also, however, stand by my statement (opinion) that I think people dealing with PMDD should consider not having children. It seems that children brought up into traumatic households have a higher likelihood of developing cPTSD or at least modeling their future relationships on the relationships they saw as normal. Whether cPTSD contributes to PMDD is not proven, but there are theories suggesting it... I think bringing a child into a household that cannot provide stability, love, etc is a selfish choice that further perpetuates instability as they eventually become adults with their own relationships.

I truly hope that you and your partner are able to figure out what works for both of you and that neither of you have to live with upsets, anger, walking on eggshells, etc. I have nothing but love and support for everyone on all sides of these partnerships (including the potential children that may be introduced to it against their will).

doblador_de_tierra
Oh man OP I was with you until you doubled down on the children piece…I grew up in an abusive household, with the primary aggressor being my father. He suffered from PTSD and depression, do you also suggest people that suffer from ANY mental health should not have kids? Because I can tell you my father sure as hell shouldn't have— actually my fathers aggression is deeper than mine has ever been and it has dramatically impacted my life.

Also I'm actually a nanny funny enough, I am ironically great with children despite suffering from PMDD. I think you have read a little too into the venting comments and have generalized that all women with PMDD aren't good with children because we can't get a handle on our PMDD? My kiddo loves me, and I would NEVER do anything to cause him harm— psychological or physical. That is why I stress treatment and therapy, you can live a normal life and yes, have kids and be a kind and present guardian despite having PMDD. Idk you really really lost me as a man suggesting women who suffer from PMDD shouldn't have children— and I hope you reflect. You suggesting those children are then inadvertently always going to suffer? My dude by that logic, people with ANY mental instability shouldn't have children…something just feels really off about how adamantly and ignorantly you are advocating and telling people with uterus' to not have children despite knowing having no actual actual research on the suffering of children with parents with PMDD. Also you said it all, this is a space to vent so you will find the worst case scenarios here and I want you to be open to the fact that we can indeed be great, gentle and loving care takers so long as we are taking care of ourselves through medical intervention and self compassion

dontwakethellama OP
I fully acknowledge that it is only my opinion and that everyone gets to make their own decisions on the topic.

I don't suggest that there is no value of life from children raised in that either. Simply ask yourself if you feel that growing up with a father with PTSD and depression, which then turned into you having cPTSD and PMDD, was a great experience. Why should a child be brought into a world like that?

You say that you would never do anything psychologically or physically damaging to your child... And most people with PMDD would say that they wouldn't do it to their loving partner either... Yet they do. And if one CAN control it to make sure they aren't doing anything directly to their child, why can't they use that same control to not take it out on their partner? Another level to this is what I mentioned about children modeling the relationships of their parents... Parents having seething arguments is not a great environment for those children either. If this is not connecting, it is highly possible that you have not experienced the level of PMDD that many of us have. It may have been awful and required lots of work... But it still doesn't sound like the uncontrollable beast that loses all sense of reasoning that I mentioned.

Why is my point about having children such a hard sticking point for you? I am coming at this from a childfree by choice person's POV. I looked at my situation in life and didn't feel like it would be great to bring a child into it. If you are inferring that I am saying "anyone with PMDD is a bad parent" or some version of that, I could see why that would be upsetting... That is not what I am saying though. I'm not even saying "every child that grows up with a parent with PMDD is doomed to have a terrible life" or any version of that. I'm simply saying that if the PMDD is so bad that people are coming to this sub, they may want to take a look at if it's a good option for them and not to just have kids because that's what society expects. It may take being explicitly honest with one's self as to whether it's actually a good idea.

doblador_de_tierra
Also every single child brought into this world is brought into it again at their will, some will be born to abusive parents and some will be born to wonderful parents, and we have just lost the ability to make that choice in this country anyways. I am so sorry that your experience has been so extremely negative that it has really tainted your perspective on the wonderful life we can provide kiddos in spite of the daily challenges we face. You are right, the people that are not taking accountability should seriously consider not bringing a child into that environment, I have seen posts here that absolutely validate

that. I also don't think you should lump all sufferers to that and relegate us to be people who can never provide enough stability or kindness to bring up wonderful, whole kiddos in this world— a little more food for thought.

> dontwakethellama OP
> I completely agree with you. There are degrees of this I'm sure. The degree to which I was speaking was the one I'm familiar with and once that gets repeated here and in the PMDD sub as well.... Extreme, hostile, evil.
>
> You're right, we don't get to choose if we get brought into the world. We do, however, get to choose if we bring someone into the world. If I barely had money to survive, I might want to reconsider having children. It would be nice if abusive parents had the foresight to reconsider their choice before having a child. If I had a high likelihood of passing on some debilitating genetic disease to a child, I might want to reconsider that choice.
>
> I don't say that none of these children should be born... I think that people need to consider those things seriously prior to having children. Having a child because you want one despite knowing the child has a high likelihood of suffering is selfish. It's biological, sure... There's the instinct of wanting to procreate that acts without reason. I'm asking to consider bringing reason to that conversation.

doblador_de_tierra
Ok this is much more helpful since you have elaborated, yes I did interpret what you said as anyone with PMDD is going to inherently be a terrible parent, which is probably why I got so defensive. I am also saying this from the POV of an early 30s woman who suffered without knowing to years, I think if you would have met me at say 21, I would perfectly fit the extremity of the symptoms, including lashing out, suicidal ideation to the point of planning it out, extreme depression, etc. I was straight up unapproachable and that is a lonely, sad life to live. I still suffer from extreme mood fluctuations, but my partner and I have learned how to handle those moments, give each other space and we are not always perfect, but at least we try. I have 1,000% had second thoughts of starting a family for many reasons, and most of them being it's very hard to find a non-selfish reason to bring a child into this world in the first place. And you are SO right about the fact that some sufferers lack so much access (or will) to treatment, that it really is a terrible idea to bring that child into

the world. I hope the people who have come here with the worst case scenarios really seek the support they need, and leave their partners if it is a straight up toxic and problematic relationship. And I also hope those that are holding out for their partners know that there is hope, and it might take a really long time to finally realize what is going on, address it, but once we have the tools, we can owe it to ourselves and our partners to try as damn hard as we can. And to be clear, the kiddo I nanny can ABSOLUTELY trigger me, especially in those couple of weeks leading up to my period. But there are strategies and appropriate coping mechanisms for those moments, so I can ensure both his emotional well being and mine. I am so glad we both kept replying and didn't disengage! I think my main issue was mostly the way you were communicating in that last part, which you totally recognized, and again I thought you were saying every single person with PMDD is doomed to be an awful abusive parents and that none of us should even think of starting families. I felt your genuine attempt to open up a sensitive conversation for sufferers so I just wanted to suggest how some of the ways you worded things could immediately cause a defensive reaction and not produce the conversation we both thing is so important to have! I really have appreciated your perspective, and also just to say, my diagnosis is actually medically official! So I do suffer AND I also want to offer hope— because this is so frustrating to deal with for all parties involved. Wishing you well OP, and thank you for continuing to genuinely engage!

SeaworthinessNo9563 December 18, 2024
I feel like my partner has PMDD and ADHD after doing tons of research and observing her behaviour for the past 7 years. How do you tell someone who's in complete denial that they could be suffering without making them feel attacked?

I've found myself apologizing and taking all the accountability for 7 years just to avoid any sort of blow out because the experiences I've had have been extreme. I've never received an apology, nor any sort of accountability and I've been blamed for ruining her life the entire time. We could be completely fine and having the best time and then something switches and I don't know who she becomes, panic attacks, verbal abuse, physical abuse. When I step away she uses that as an excuse to hurdle more verbal abuse m, when I'm back she ends up saying I just left her to suffer by herself and then that becomes part of the problem.

I'm struggling to navigate these issues with her as I've absorbed all the blame for years and years and ultimately I now have myself to blame for this mess.

I know it's not personal, well I don't. But I give the situation the benefit of the doubt, however where I suffer the most is that there's zero awareness and accountability from her. So I've always felt like I owe her because I've wronged her and that's the narrative in the relationship.

dontwakethellama OP
I'll give you a little tough love here:
You think that by apologizing and taking accountability for all the problems is helping, but it isn't. You are enabling her behavior. You need to have boundaries and she needs to respect them.

You HAVE to talk these through when everything is good. You need to bring all of it up while things are going well even if you are afraid that it will end in a fight... Learn ways of opening these conversations in a constructive way.

I am hearing some classic "nice guy" and codependency in your situation... Something that is common in these relationships. This is where you can grow and help lead the relationship out of the typical path. You both have to be on board for it. If she is not willing to work with you on it, then there is nothing you can do... Either choose to continue and accept the abuse, or remove yourself from the situation.

This all applies whether she has PMDD or not. Her being abusive is not acceptable. You must respect yourself more than the memory of what the relationship used to be. Hopefully she will be open to reading about PMDD and talking to a doctor about it to know for sure.
Best of luck to you in all of this.

The original post at the sub.[19]

---

19 https://www.reddit.com/r/PMDDpartners/comments/1b6k2i7

Core Posts

My practice was if I wrote the same comment five or more times I would consider turning that comment into a section of the wiki or a post so I wouldn't have to repeat myself ... as much. A majority of the wiki is in the previous sections. These are my most referenced posts.

Science has shown the best way to deal with anger,
anybody's anger, is to take a time out.

You're going to be wrong no matter what you do,
so you may as well do what's right.

It's hard to hear anything when you're being yelled at.

Unenforced boundaries are just suggestions.

Fundamentally PMDD is chemistry.
Will power and good intentions will only get you so far.

Why is this not Common Knowledge?

(Taking a time out)

Phew-ThatWasClose - August 4, 2024

OOOOOH. I get soooooo angry!

I attend a group anger zoom through my health care provider to try and work on my anger around PMDD and the lost years and the misplaced blame and etc. It's not going very well because it's mostly about how to *control or manage* your anger. My anger is under control, but ever present. I want to get rid of it. I didn't used to feel this way. I want to feel peace and calm and, maybe happiness? I'm thinking probably drugs.

Not the point. Point is the leader of the zoom is a soft spoken kinda goofy guy who just presents this information with little fanfare and I go away and think about it and it blows me away. This is what he told us last week.

When you get angry, when anyone gets angry, the adrenaline spikes and you're in survival mode. When that happens your body shifts focus into fight or flight. If it's a lion on the Serengeti you'll pick flight. If it's an obnoxious drunk you may pick fight. Especially if you are also drunk and you can soooo totally take that guy.

Also not the point. Point is when that adrenaline spikes your pre-frontal cortex *starts to shut down*. That's the part of the brain responsible for rational decision making. That part *shuts down* within about *two minutes* and after the pre-frontal cortex shuts down you are *no longer capable* of rational decision making.

That makes sense because survival is paramount and everything else is secondary. One major thing that suddenly becomes less important once the pre-frontal cortex shuts down is consequences. Without a functioning pre-frontal cortex you no longer have any consideration for, *or even a concept of*, consequences.

ALSO, as if that weren't enough, you lose about 30 IQ points. As my son put it "Oh, so I'd have average intelligence." and I responded "Yes, but still above average arrogance." For the rest of us we become imbeciles. 100 is average. People with 70 IQ need velcro shoes. When you are in the thick of it you are functionally a moron.

For me that's how I know I'm in the thick of it. I get brain fog and nothing makes sense anymore. To be fair she's not making sense anyway because she's also lost 30 IQ points. The implications for this community are vast.

We frequently lament "why doesn't she know?" or "why doesn't she remember?" and the common response is "it's the Dysphoria." But that's only part of it. To be honest dysphoria is just fancy for depressed and confused. The real problem is she's an idiot, and so are we. Just two simpletons screaming at each other.

And **THAT** is why we keep saying "walk away". As soon as you become aware it's one of *those* conversations tell her you love her, you'll talk about it next week, but not right now, and Walk Away!! You have two minutes. Less as you've already noticed the early warning signs. If you can't get away make the conscious decision to grey rock and stick to it. NOTHING will help, EVERYTHING will make it worse.

There have been times when I have literally run out of the house because I knew if I stayed one more second I'd respond and chaos would ensue. Now I know why.

ETA: The followup to this post appears <u>here</u> (p.114).

> PadreDeBlas
> "I'm thinking probably drugs"
>
> Have you tried sports?
>
> The gym isn't my happy place, it's my angry place, where I let those feelings drain out of my pores.
>
> Love you bud, keep doing the good work!
>
>> Phew-ThatWasClose OP
>> 😁 Already grew the mushrooms. But your idea is good too.
>>
>>> PadreDeBlas
>>> Wait till you combine them, oh boy! Micro dosing can be enjoyable on the ski slope, the golf course (once hit a disc golf ace while on 0.3g of PE after making a 100' putt) or on your bike, etc, etc. Smoking weed and lifting is somehow relaxing.
>
> SantoriniBisque
> This is a great post. It makes me wish I could go back and rethink some of my choices with her. Not that it would have prevented different fights.

I think about that sometimes though. What if you had a time machine and could go and stop the fights you knew were coming. I still don't think it will prevent the inevitable outcome in the end. She would still find a way to battle with you or find a fault. There were many times she had no ammo to come at me and the dysphoria still fabricated ideas to attack me.

Walking away is the only way. Sadly this time I walked away for the last time

HusbandofPMDD
Sorry about this. Deep breaths.

That said, I find it helpful to try post processing once I've calmed down and then address the root. Anger is the emotion you feel after you cognitively feel like you're experiencing injustice (perceived or real). Figuring out how to make peace about the perceived injustice and learning tools to choose other coping mechanism is what actually will make a difference.

I'm sure you know this, but it's what I find measured success with

> Phew-ThatWasClose OP
> Making peace with a perceived injustice is a huge stumbling block for me and, I'm sure, others. As I said my resident anger ruminates on the lost years, the false accusations, the skewed world view, and the lack of any ownership. We're out of that now, and she has apologized profusely, but there's still an undercurrent of both-siderism that grates like a pebble in your shoe.
>
> Deep Breaths. Always a good idea.
>
> > HusbandofPMDD
> > I feel ya. I think we're all taking turns experiencing the pain and then recovering to coach someone else. Today you, tomorrow me!

SAOCORE
Lol, something in the post starting with 'I get soooo angry' told me this is likely not a pmdd 'partner'

Mugatu-Utagum

30 IQ points is very specific. Do you have a link to this data?

Phew-ThatWasClose OP
I do not. I was just parroting what the guy with the degree said. I found a Psychology Today article that said 10-15 points but not 30. I will ask the group lead next chance.

Mugatu-Utagum
And are you stating this applies to the effects of PMDD on both partners, or more specifically what happens during any given survival/fight or flight/trauma response?

Phew-ThatWasClose OP
It's true for any situation that triggers a fight or flight response. It's appropriate, and may save your life, on the Serengeti. Interacting with a your life partner … not so much.

If rage is a symptom she struggles with she's already compromised and trying to push your buttons. She has no concept of the consequences. She's not thinking rationally. Engaging will accomplish nothing at that point except give her more opportunity to push more buttons. If she succeeds then you join the madness and insanity wins the day.

We all already knew this empirically. Now we know why. And we have a measure of the urgency. You have two minutes. I'll try to find a source for that fun fact as well. :)

Phew-ThatWasClose OP August 8, 2024
My Group Lead said it came from Dr. Ross Greene who is a child psychologist at Harvard. He wrote a book titled The Explosive Child and has pioneered the "Collaborative Proactive Solutions" (CPS) model for working with kids who have regulation challenges and explosive tempers.

Technically it's "up to 30" IQ points lost when the prefrontal cortex (PFC) shuts down. The main problem arises when adults try to discipline kids who have no control. The idea behind CPS is the kids would regulate if they could, they just don't know how. So by talking about it, instead of disciplining and punishing, you create a better outcome.

It all seems very familiar.

Mugatu-Utagum August 15, 2024
Interesting stuff, thank you for sharing. Although my wife has PMDD, her symptoms can and often do exceed "luteal" phase - I suspect she also has chronic PTSD. Both PTSD and PMDD have very similar symptoms, so when she's PMDDing it's on top of whatever already exists. But I also feel like that explains what I see, her PFC shut down - if she's not anxious or panicked or overstimulated, she's lethargic and unpleasant. It's like she's almost always in fight or flight. She just got brain scans done so in a couple weeks she will be diagnosed based off physical, tangible evidence and not just symptoms. After all this time, I've got to admit I'm pretty excited to finally know what has been ailing her. I'm tempted to get my own brain scans done after the insanity and depths this has played a part in bringing me to.

SpaceYeastFeast
Walking say / gray rock is the best approach. If she is already upset in luteal, when you speak there is a very good chance it will sound offensive to her, or not supportive enough. That's if you want to stay for love , children or are stuck for financial reasons. If none of those things apply then run as fast as you can.

chilllpill
When we get to that point and I try to walk away, I am told I'm conflict avoidant. If I come back and things only got worse since she feels rejected because I triggered her Rejection Sensitivity Dysphoria, which then triggers her suicidal ideation. Things really start getting dangerous, and if I leave during SI, it triggers her abandonment wound, which becomes the narrative for the next month. "How could you leave me during my most critical time of need. You don't care about my life!" Compound this with having a small kid, and my leaving and taking him with me triggers her feeling of shame, or that I'm using him as a shield to avoid more tough conversations. Just leaving seems so easy…but it isn't!

Phew-ThatWasClose OP
Absolutely it's hard. I like the saying "You're going to be wrong no matter what you do. So you might as well do what's right." It sounds trite because it is. But it highlights the most important thing. What is best for the kid?

What is best for the kid is two functional parents. Second best is one functional parent. Right now the kid has no functional parents because the PMDD rules them both. She's going to say what she's going to say.

If it's not one thing it's another. RSD and abandonment wounds and shame and using SI as a tactic … it's all just manipulation and, ultimately, it's just Abuse.

You *are* conflict avoidant. Of course you are. Why wouldn't you be? There's nothing but conflict in that conflict. It won't be resolved. She won't "get it out of her system." There's just pain and misery and a spiral of doom. Avoid that. It's Horrible. It's Abuse.

Tolerating abuse is not support. Letting the PMDD control the narrative, and thereby control your lives, benefits no one. Talk about it during follicular. Set the expectation that you will be leaving, and taking the kid, when the abuse starts. Not forever, 20 minutes is enough to disrupt the spiral. Then come back and *don't talk about it*.

Also during follicular come up with a plan to avoid that happening in the first place. What does she need during luteal to help her manage the symptoms. Specifically. Not "Be supportive." or "Don't trigger me." but specific concrete things each of you can do to make that time less of a struggle. Does she need food? a bath? a cold plunge? an SSRI? You to do the laundry? You to take the kid so she can veg? Make a plan. Write it on paper. Magnet it to the fridge.

None of it is easy. But it becomes less difficult over time.

ManufacturerLevel488 August 18, 2024
Everything about this minus the kid is my experience with walking away too. I can relate so much.

You haven't discovered a solution to this in the last 11 days have you? 😬

> chilllpill
> No solution, but leaving the room/home does remove you and her from abuse and harm. So do it!
>
> > ManufacturerLevel488
> > Need to dust off my courage!

workaccount1338 January 19, 2025
commenting to save this thread. Wow.

OddAd667 July 1, 2025
Comment for reference

The original post on the sub.[1]

---

1   https://www.reddit.com/r/PMDDpartners/comments/1ek4rwc

Three Simple Steps To Managing Your Anger.

Phew-ThatWasClose - September 8, 2024

I'm in this zoom group through my health care that is intended to help with anger management. In my case my ex is in menopause so the PMDD years are behind us. But I still have a lot of residual anger around the lost years and the history of abuse and the triggers that abuse created. And we're still co-parenting two incredible kids so it's work to avoid those triggers.

For others I imagine there are similar issues in real time. And certainly women with PMDD, who experience rage as a symptom, might benefit from a little anger management. So here's the deal. You fill out this form (p.296), you read the form aloud once a day for thirty days, then you're cured. Easy peasy.

The group lead likes to point out that they need to be three *simple* steps because when you are activated you are an idiot (p.107).

Step 1: Notice. This is the hardest step. We bop through our life and we generally don't notice what's going on because much of life is automatic habit. Same is true of anger. We notice when we are angry, but few of us notice when we are becoming angry. Part of the problem is becoming angry happens quickly. It only takes about two minutes for the pre-frontal cortex to *shut down* and then it's too late. So you have two minutes to notice the signs and do something about it.

Reflect on what those signs are. Think back to just before you got angry. What are your triggers? For me I can't stand catastrophising. I hate the disgusted facial expressions and the gag/ick/eww noises. I write these long posts and comments but I don't actually talk very much so when I do have something to say I hate being interrupted. I especially hate being interrupted and having the conversation hijacked and taken to a disastrous place I totally was never going and then having that wack-a-doo notion attributed to me. Not what I said. Not what I was going to say. Not even remotely what I ever even came close to thinking.

Think back to how your body feels just before you get angry. For me I get a shortness of breath, a brain fog, a pit in my stomach, I start to scan the room (looking for the exit?), I start to drum, my body temperature rises, I feel flushed. Think about the cliches. "He saw red" - I get tunnel vision. "It was like a gut punch" - mine is more twisted in knots. "There was steam coming out his ears" - no steam but I definitely feel like my brain is getting warm.

What is your body actually doing? Does your spine straighten? Do you get sewing machine leg? Do your shoulders tense up? Do you drum like I do? Does your facial expression change? Can you feel your eyes glaze over? Does your voice change pitch or timbre?

Think about all that and write your signals down on the handout (p.296).

Step 2: Separate and Calm. This is the easiest and most important step. Once you have identified the signals you have less than two minutes to GTFO. Taking a time out is the number one doctor recommended method for avoiding a cataclysmic battle of the Kaiju. You know from experience that nothing good will come from sticking around. You need to leave, and leave now! Tell her you love her, and you'll be back, but GO!

And go do something calming or some self care or something to burn off the energy or all of that. And while you're calming yourself down she is calming herself down (because she filled out one of these too) and you can meet up again in an hour. Bring froyo.

Step 3: Plan and Assert. During the calm down period you also start to think about why you were getting angry in the first place. Something was threatening something you value. What was that all about? How can you best express your concerns and needs in an assertive but respectful and caring way? The buzzwords are: "Bold", "Direct", "Respectful", and "Clear".

Standard advice is to use "I" statements of the form "I feel __________ when you __________ because ___________ and instead I need _____________." You might rehearse. You might even write it down. For example "I feel frustrated when you interrupt because I don't feel heard or respected and instead I need you to wait for me to finish what I am saying before responding."

And that probably will **not** get you the result you hoped for. But that's not the point. The point is you kept yourself in a state of honor and integrity while asserting your concerns and needs in a bold, direct, respectful and clear way. If your concerns are ignored and your needs unmet you can deal with that when it happens and if the pattern continues you make a decision.

But here is where we diverge from the standard scheme. A lot of Step 3 is irrelevant to us because mostly the arguments in luteal are just nonsense. Normally therapists would have you reconvene after the calm down but for us, we know re-engaging during luteal is ill advised. You may well write down your "I" statement and bring it up a week later, at your strategy meeting during follicular. But then you just note that that happened, and what can we do to prevent that next luteal?

Step 4: Talk to her about Step 1. Because the real trick is if she can notice her own signals and redirect herself without lashing out at her loved ones. Many of you have said *you* notice her signals. A change in intonation, phrases she starts to use, mannerisms. Is that something she can become aware of. It could be something as simple as wanting to use the phrase "You always ..." or noticing that you breath really loud or realizing that she asked you to make her a cup of tea *five minutes ago* and she *still* has no tea! Can she catch herself and storm out the door screaming "I HAVE TO GO!   FOR A WALK!!   NOW!!!" instead.

But fill out the form (p.296) then read it out loud, enunciating in a clear voice, once a day for thirty days. That is supposed to bring it to top of mind when the need arises and make it easier to interrupt the negative spiral before it gets out of control. Meet back here in 31 days and we'll all compare notes.

AvalonTeals
Thank you so much for sharing this resource!

workaccount1338

.

OddAd667 July 1, 2025
Wish i could have found this earlier, i love the humour of I AM GOING FOR A WALK NOW!!!!!!

The original post on the sub.[2]

There is a pdf of the form[3] online.

---

2   https://www.reddit.com/r/PMDDpartners/comments/1fboy94
3   https://drive.google.com/file/d/1W8zTYb7p8KjRCKxiuiuWTjevgTvBnxNH/view

Do. Not. Apologize.

Phew-ThatWasClose August 23, 2024

I've seen an uptick in comments that say "no matter how much I try to reassure her and apologize she still …"

I get it. I've been in the cross-hairs. You're the worst person since Andrew Tate. You're a horrible father and a worse husband. You're abusive and disrespectful. My ex once told me I was "just like Trump" which backfired when I laughed. But it's incessant and grating and she seemingly has infinite capacity. You just want it to stop any way possible. You'll agree to anything at that point just to *make it stop*. But don't. Because it won't. And now it's worse.

You're wrong no matter what you do so you might as well do what's right. You can't wait it out. Sometimes you may have to which is where greyrocking comes in, but settle in cause the PMDD has a lot to talk about. And if the PMDD runs out of things to say it'll just circle back and start over. What I used to do is I used to say "Please Stop". And I would say that over and over like a mantra. And I did that for two years.

So the temptation is to give her what she says she wants. She says she wants to be heard and validated. Except you didn't do the thing she says you did. You weren't dismissive. You weren't disrespectful. You weren't selfish. You weren't uncaring. She may well have perceived it that way but her perception is skewed. And probably you are sorry she feels that way but you didn't do what she says you did and you certainly didn't intend what she says you intended.

So okay. Maybe apologize. Once. "Oh, sorry if it came across that way. That's never what I intended." And that's it. One and done. Grown ups, who are not compromised, can accept that and move on. If she insists *this offense* is the worst thing since the Dobbs decision you need to stop. She's in luteal. She is literally not rational. The rage overrides and no amount of apologizing is going to make it stop.

What apologizing does do, however, is it makes everything **true**. You did do the horrible thing else why would you apologize? And why would you apologize *so much*? And while the dysphoria may have her forget the rage she will remember that you did something awful and she *had to* yell at you to get you to apologize. That pattern becomes normalized and if it repeats cycle after cycle pretty soon it's a habit and it doesn't even have to be luteal anymore.

You can't wait it out and you can't smooth it over. Arguing just makes it worse. What can you do? If the love of your life has PMDD, and one of her symptoms is inconsolable rage, the best thing you can do *for everybody* is don't be there. Take a walk, go to the gym, go get a froyo. Be elsewhere for an hour.

The obvious benefit to you is you don't get berated and belittled. Maybe you're strong and you can take it. Doesn't matter. Your brain takes it in. The woman you love thinks you're horrid. Plus it's wasting your time, energy and resource for no benefit to anyone. It's not helping her at all.

With you there the rage has a target. The longer you are there the longer the rage has a target. The rage will not flame out. The rage will just spiral into more and bigger rage. The longer you are there the worse your perceived infraction becomes and the PMDD convinces her it's all real. **Words have power.** The more she repeats it, out loud, the truer it becomes.

With you gone the rage has no target. Nothing to rage at. She may scream. She may stim and stomp her feet and think you're awful for leaving in the middle of a "conversation". But ultimately, and shortly, the rage does fade into fleh. And probably she'll turn inward and feel terrible about everything and cry for hours. But she's not doing any damage, she won't be ashamed or defensive later, and she won't normalize the lies her PMDD is telling her about you.

Then, during follicular, you don't have to spend all your time recovering. Instead you can spend time working to mitigate the symptoms for next time and … celebrating the reasons you fell in love in the first place.

Dependent-Expert-407
Thanks for sharing! I completely resonate with this.

iaamanthony
Thank you for saying this! I really needed to hear it today.

Baloneous_V
It's a battlefield littered with "nice guys". Its the perfect killing grounds for men that were raised to honor and respect women, no matter what and to always be responsible for the effect your behavior has on others.

I agree with this post 100%

I've used this stage of life to really mature emotionally and only look at what I can control in my life. I've got PMDD to thank for keeping me on my toes psychologically and habitually and its given me an extra layer of armor and a bag of tools to face all kinds of shit in life that really doesn't matter as much as I once thought.

I've got a motto of STFU for myself when I want to rage and that includes apologies 💀

> PadreDeBlas
> "Never miss an opportunity to STFU."
>
> I'm with you. We've hardened ourselves through constant use of relationship survival skills. We're playing marriage on hard mode. Everything else in my life, professionally, socially, as a father, is easy by comparison as if it were, pardon the term, beginner mode.
>
>> TalentIntel
>> Well. This put my life in perspective - I constantly question myself. How is everything else great. It's on difficult mode.

PadreDeBlas
Damn Phew, I've never felt so heard and seen. Thanks for this!

Edit to add: I'm going to get a froyo after the gym.

runemforit
Great practical advice, thanks for sharing

RDG3PO
💯 I apologized for so many things I had no control over that I started to gaslight myself. Lasting damage.

> PieceKind2819
> Aka erosion of self. ;)

HusbandofPMDD
I think it's nuanced. You need to take ownership of what is yours (I shouldn't have engaged, I shouldn't have raised my voice, that was sarcastic), while being clear that you're not owning her behaviours. You will get into an unhealthy state if you blanket say sorry, and she will get frustrated by your inability to accurately state what you did wrong.

Too often apologies in PMDD relationships are partners trying to stop the conflict and it's just codependency. As OP said, say your bit and walk away.

While text is not a healthy form of communication for a healthy relationship, text is very effective during luteal as it can't be twisted or misrepresented. Also, it separates you 1 layer from an emotional response. For these reasons use text in high tension times.

> GetTheLead_Out
> The one caveat to text is there can't be a text battle. Because that can get really, really bad. But brief, to the point, then disengage.
>
> I live with my brother. If I act crazy (anyone who sees my comments know I isolate like a master so it's rare that people see the crazy), I will send a quick text to debrief. Then we discuss briefly, and no more texts. also think saying "I'm going on do not disturb for the next 2 hours so I can work (nap, decompress, hike, whatever)" is wise.
>
> Apparently it makes people feel abandoned, but I think if you can state it clearly that you won't be available it allows both to decompress alone without desiring to engage more.
>
> > HusbandofPMDD
> > Good point

blue_baphomet
Thank you!

DaneDad78
Thank you

EtoileNoirr
This post resonates

__d_o_o_d__
It's like you're in my head!

Federal-Stomach-2380
I have PMDD and I'm grateful it's the suicidal crying type and not the hostile type. Can't imagine acting this way with my gf

undercuv-bruv
I didn't read past the first sentence man since i don't wanna feel it again but i hope you're OK my brother... and really all my broken bros and sisters out there too.. The suffering is too much

Visual-Ratio-3672
Well said, my partner get's so worked up about me owning and apologizing for anything. Been taking so much shit for so many years. Well no more.

boopskittlybop
Damn...it's so real. I've definitely said some hurtful stuff in the heat of the fights that I have really needed to apologize for but I agree. I wish I would have set boundaries more rather than do the codependent apologizing to assuage the situation OR let pmdd and the emotional exhaustion of it control me. Apologizing for things I was not sorry for and didn't agree with only made it worse and then when I addressed the ways I took too much responsibility in the past, it was used against me to say I wasn't taking responsibility 😵 🙇 . What a great post.

obsoado
Thanks for the post ! It's accurate, as long as no one uses it to justify harmful behaviors. PMDD is real, but dysfunctional relationships are a separate issue imo

TalentIntel
I apologize soooo much. Yesterday I was told I am just like her ex - her ex husband who caused all of her trauma and ptsd. Then belittled me to our family by telling them I don't make any money and don't pay for anything. She said I don't respect her almost every day

Yet she is unemployed and I pay for everything. I still apologized.

I always apologize. I feel gross after

EitherAccountant6736

I am new to the sub, but this is near identical to my situation.

My recent partner's previous relationship was with someone with npd and the result was trauma and ptsd.

She claims that the chaos that we experience is new to our relationship, but I find it hard to believe that some of her patterns and behaviors didn't come out in her past.

Was the previous guy just like us, and we will be the villain for the next person?

Requiascat April 11, 2025
I just found this sub after being on Reddit for 13 years. My partner and I have been together for 8 and have been through the ups and downs of her trying all sorts of different things to combat this. She was misdiagnosed with Bi-polar 1 and 2 and has gone through I dont know how many other drugs and self-medication until she tried Yas.

Yas worked for a while but started destroying her liver. Now we're back to square one and

I've been dreading the eventual shift to hating me again and threatening to leave.

We went to bed last night after having a good day and this morning after waking up she hates me again and can't wait to leave me. I didn't do anything, nothing changed. I'm just the villian again.

She has a doctor's appointment Tuesday to maybe try one last alternative before surgery as a last resort.

Reading these comments makes me feel so validated about all of this. I've been wondering if maybe I'm delusional and she's right about me. I've apologized for everthing just to make it stop, to end the abuse and get on with providing for my family.

I feel like I've been seen for the first time just reading everybody's experiences.

So happy I found this place.

Phew-ThatWasClose OP
Welcome.

I'm curious how you stumbled on this 8 month old thread. Surely you didn't read down to this point.

I had not heard of Yaz messing with livers. That sucks. But at least she is open to meds which sometimes an uphill battle around here. Bipolar is a common misdiagnosis. So did they give her an SSRI? If not a low dose intermittent SSRI (p.26) is recommended for PMDD.

I get the frustration but surgery comes with it's own set of issues. HRT can be tricky.

Literally anything else (p.284) is a better option. One alternative many don't think of is Acupuncture[4].

She's wrong about you. You're not the villain. PMDD is the villain.

> Requiascat
> I sorted by Top Posts of All Time and the title grabbed me by the bollocks lol
>
> SSRIs tend to worsen her symptoms. She has PCOS *and* PMDD. It's like her ovaries have no schedule and are cranked to 11 without medical intervention.
>
> Tuesday we go to her gyno and she wants to explore anti-androgens and the low-dose intermittent SSRIs. If they dont work surgery is basically her only option at this point.
>
> Yas can really screw with the liver but it's a very rare side-effect that had us in the emergency room a couple times after she had been on it for a few months. One isn't necessarily supposed to feel pain in their liver, but she did and it was severe enough to warrant a couple trips before trial, error, and a battery of tests confirmed it was the Yas.
>
> I know I'm not the villian, but it can be easy to think, "…maybe *I'm* the one that's fucked up…". But I'm a 13 years sober alcoholic—if anyone in this relationship knows how to take a personal inventory and be reflective about their behavior it's me.
>
> Thanks for reading me vent. I'm so glad I found this sub. I was searching for support groups at work and stumbled onto this sub. Glad to be here.

---

4   http://www.reddit.com/r/PMDD/comments/1csqbaj

> Phew-ThatWasClose OP
> That's hilarious. :)
>
> For PMDD SSRI's can be used *as needed*. So that might be a good fit for one with irregular cycles. There are folks on the other sub[5] that also have PCOS so run a search over there. Sounds like she's done her research though.
>
> I hear you. I spent years wondering if she might have a point. I am also not the villain, despite what some might say. Surprise surprise - I wrote about it[6]. :)
>
> Good luck on Tuesday.

> Nrock49 April 30, 2025
> Literally same. Been on reddit for years, been together for 8, just joined sub and am so happy to know I'm not alone.

>> Requiascat
>> You truly are not alone friend. It's really refreshing, in a weird way I guess, to hear other folks going through the same shit. Kinda like a recover hall/support group lol

MiNiX97 June 29, 2025
I cannot like this enough. It is so incredibly spot on. I've been lurking this sub for quite a while. I'm eventually going to have to bring up with her that I think she has PMDD, so that when I finally muster the courage to just walk away during The Rage, she will know that I'm doing it because of PMDD and not just because I'm walking out on her (which would only make the relationship worse I think). Once she is aware, then walking out becomes an option because I can later say "I walked out because that was our pre-planned response to The Rage."

> Phew-ThatWasClose OP
> Consider writing your plan down (p.58) and posting it on the fridge. Instead of just "I'm taking a time out when you rage" you can build in safeguards to help prevent it happening, and support for both of you to stay on track during luteal. It's like I always say sometimes. Luteal is a lot less chaotic, and a lot more manageable, when it's scripted. :)

The original post on the sub.[7]

---

5   http://www.reddit.com/r/PMDD/search/?q=pcos
6   http://www.reddit.com/r/PMDDpartners/comments/1hqbmln/comment/m4oe2nd
7   https://www.reddit.com/r/PMDDpartners/comments/1ezeqsa

You are the Lion!

Phew-ThatWasClose - January 26, 2025

In the past I have written about the adrenaline spike, the fight or flight response, the 30 point slide, and the Pre-frontal Cortex shutdown. That post is here (p.107). The TL;DR is *walk away.* Once you are aware it is one of *those* conversations just walk away. She'll get mad at you for abandoning her or disrespecting or invalidating or whatever, but she's going to be mad at you anyway and she will be less mad, for less time, if you're not there.

This is why: You are the Lion.

The PMDD has convinced her that you are a threat to something she cares about. That "something she cares about" may even be you. Maybe the PMDD has convinced her you're going to leave her. Maybe the PMDD has convinced her your views on fluoridated water mean you don't care about the kids health. Maybe the PMDD has convinced her you doing all the dishes save the one you left to soak is proof you never do anything to help out around here.

It doesn't have to make sense. The PMDD can be very convincing and it convinces her something she cares about is being threatened *by you.* That triggers the fight or flight response and the PMDD chooses fight. She might even seek you out and start baiting because you are a threat and the PMDD needs to fight you. And once the adrenaline spikes, the fight or flight kicks in, and the PFC *shuts down* nothing else matters until the threat is neutralized.

This is why apologies dont work (p.117). Can you imagine a Lion saying "I'm sorry I didn't do the vacuuming last Tuesday." It's still a Lion. Placating doesn't work. Can you imagine a Lion saying "Try not to worry, it'll be okay." It's still a Lion. Greyrocking doesn't even work. Greyrocking just prolongs the episode because a Lion staring off into the distance not saying anything is *still a Lion*!

It's a metaphor, but not *just* a metaphor. The PMDD says there really really is a threat and with the PFC shut down the brain does not know the difference between dishes not being done and a Lion. That's not me being dramatic. I checked with my therapist. There have been studies. You need to leave. Walk away.

Even if she sought you out, you have to leave because she cannot. Just to the other room. Just for half an hour. Long enough for the PFC to come back on line. Sometimes I just walk to the kitchen to refill my water, then walk back to my room and close the door. There, the Lion is behind a closed door. Nothing to worry about.

Sometimes you may need to leave the house. Go get a froyo. Bring her back one. She'll need one after that scary episode with the Lion.

8 https://www.reddit.com/r/PMDDpartners/comments/1iaqmxl

The original post on the sub.[8]

---

8 https://www.reddit.com/r/PMDDpartners/comments/1iaqmxl

Boundaries

Phew-ThatWasClose - June 27, 2025
A while back someone commented that unenforced boundaries are just suggestions and I thought "smarmy asshole". But it stuck with me and after a bit I realized he was right. All that time I spent screaming "GET THE FUCK AWAY FROM ME!" I wasn't actually doing enough to get the fuck away from her.

People talk about setting boundaries and then they talk about how, during luteal, those boundary conditions get thrown out the window. I've been reminded, and had a couple times this week where I reminded others, that they're not *her* boundaries, they're yours. Prevailing thought seems to be that you get together during follicular and discuss, and say things like "Okay, this is the line, do not cross this line." Then she says "Okay, gotcha." and then luteal shows up and the PMDD crosses the line. And then you make shocked pikachu face and say "Whaaaat? But we agreed!!"

That's not the way boundaries work. They are *your* boundaries. They are you describing to yourself what you will not put up with. They are important because unless you formally *set* the boundary you're just wingin' it and reacting in the moment. That's not awful because we're with our partner. That's meant to be our safe space and we shouldn't *need* set boundaries because our *partner* wouldn't come anywhere near something like that. Which is why many of us are caught flat footed when the PMDD rage shows up and tramples all over anything resembling descent, respectful, or caring behavior.

A lot of us lose ourselves because we don't know what to do. So we ask "Please don't do that anymore." Then next luteal rolls around and *that* thing is the *first* thing the PMDD does. So that's not a boundary, that's a request.

A boundary is a description of what you will not put up with. You can share it with her, but that's not necessary. It's not rule, or a threat, or an ultimatum. It's you imposing your own self respect on yourself. "I will not be treated this way." And so, when the PMDD tries to treat you that way, you walk. "Nope, not having it." There's no bargaining. No pleading. No reasoning. Just walk. You *will not* be treated that way, so don't be.

My ex is, no surprise, the mother of my children. We all live together again and it works because she's in menopause so there's no more PMDD. There's no more affection either but she's nice enough and we have great kids. Nevertheless the lessons learned from the PMDD are still *right there*. I was reminded today that one of my boundaries is "I will not be supervised."

She has some vision about the chicken coop that entails me and the boy moving it halfway across the yard. It's a big annoying project that I didn't want to do but I'm doing it anyway because ultimately I think the kids will benefit in some small way. Today is day two of the project so I'm tired from day one, and now I'm doing all the fiddly stuff, and it's hotter than it was yesterday, and *she is hovering!* She's telling me what to do and pointing out a spot I missed and talking about next steps and <u>I start to recognize my signals</u> (p.114). So I said "will you go away?" and she said "No, absolutely not." and I put down my tools and walked. She instantly said "Okay, okay, okay, I'll leave, keep working." so I came back and she didn't bother me for the rest of the day. Still not done. :<(

Took a decade to get to this point but, as the kids say, "Ta-Frickin-Da!"

Reasonable-Weird258_
Great reminder. It is one I am actively learning, so thank you. Good luck with the coop relocation project.

tx_hempknight_
Not being supervised is going on my list. Lmao

vickrumhugo_
How do you work when walking away doesn't work, my partner will just start to scream if I walk away or become verbally abusive etc?

Phew-ThatWasClose
Walk further, walk faster. I once walked eight blocks and she was barefoot. If you won't tolerate it don't. That boundary doesn't change when she escalates. Leave the room, leave the house, leave the neighborhood. Half an hour for the PFC to come back online. If she's still raging when you return, head back out. It is not okay.

She may well rage that you're disrespectful or you don't care or you're manipulative or whatever. None of that is okay either. And don't talk about it until follicular. Then you <u>make a plan</u> (p.69) for preventing it next time.

I greyrocked for two years at one point and nothing changed. I ended up a shell and my kids learned all the wrong lessons. When I started walking things started to change. In the wrong direction at first, but I got my freedom and I got my self back. Then I was able to work to make a real difference.

chilllpill

How do you walk away when you have a small child at home? Take them with you? I've tried, and then got told for weeks how I put our child in the middle of our fight and traumatized him. Or if you walk away, what if they say "OK", lock the door, and text you to find someplace to stay, and you're stuck walking around in your pajamas while the sun is setting and it starts raining. Been there, not fun!

Phew-ThatWasClose_
More than a few times I tried to leave and she got in the car with me. Once I had the genius idea to drive to the police station but she was screaming and I only made it a block before I had to pull over and run. Once she convinced me to buy her breakfast out because she had no money, then started talking about all the garbage so I left and she followed me to my car so I walked around the mall and she followed me harping the entire time and I got back to the car and she had left her purse in the restaurant and wouldn't go in because she'd been crying and she was embarrassed so I got that for her and then she still wouldn't let me get in my car so I walked around the mall again with her following again and harping and … yeah.

Have a go bag in the car, a spare key stashed, talk to a lawyer about documenting and what counts as evidence and always remember greyrocking is a survival strategy. So if you get to that point lock up all your emotion and greyrock like a motherfucker. Deep fucking breaths.

There is no way I could ever have left with the kids. But I was also always confident she wouldn't hurt them no matter how angry she was at me. If you are not confident of that you need to work on getting out (p.56) with full custody.

Casual-Zpring-710
Spot on… I've found it only leads them to seek out smashing those boundaries during the luteal phase. "Please can you try to not slam doors, as I worry of the complaints from neighbours and the shops below." Then proceeds to smash every door shut as hard as she possibly can during this time.

jackgwynn
Thank you for the reminder; it's something I'm actively working on. Best of luck with your coop relocation project!

The original post on the sub.[9]

---

9   https://www.reddit.com/r/PMDDpartners/comments/1llq28j

Treatment is unique in multiple ways.

Phew-ThatWasClose – August 09, 2025

I read this sub and the other sub every day and try to help if I can. I get frustrated when people say things like "I've tried everything and nothing helps." or "not interested in BC or antidepressants" or "The Pill made it worse" or "had a bad experience with SSRIs a few years ago". If I'm having a bad day I might think to myself "oh well, I guess there's no hope then."

But on a better day I might think "Which SSRI at what dosage?" or "What pill? Exactly?" or "Really? Everything?" And on that day I might write a comment like this:

The DSM-5 <u>defines PMDD</u> (p.268) as any 5 of a possible 11 symptoms that create significant interference with work, school, relationships, etc. Consequently PMDD is wildly different in every instance. Moreover it is estimated PMDD is misdiagnosed in up to 40% of cases, there may be comorbidities (like Bipolar or Borderline), and there may be an underlying issue that is only unmasked during luteal (PME).

Point is <u>recommended treatment</u> (p.22) is not going to help everyone. You are the expert on you and if you're hesitant to try something that is fair. But be sure it's for the right reasons. Science based recommended treatments help *most*. And they are quite specific recommendations so don't dismiss them until you are *sure* you have tried them.

PMDD is not as well known in the medical community as one might wish. Many doctors are only dimly aware and will just throw stuff at you. It's to do with her cycle? Shut that fucker down! It's causing anxiety? Put her on an SSRI! But there is a lot more to it than that and *you* need to become the expert.

The Pill is not one thing. There are categories and varieties. Progestin Only Pills (POPs) and triphasics are **not** recommended for women with PMDD. Both these categories of birth control are adequate for preventing conception but can actually make PMDD symptoms *worse*. PMDD is an abnormal reaction to normal *changes* in hormone levels during the reproductive cycle. POPs and triphasics do nothing to prevent, and in some cases amplify, those changes.

Monophasic Combined Oral Contraceptives **are** what is <u>recommended</u> (p.22) by both RCOG and ACOG. Taken continuously monophasic COCs suppress ovulation and eliminate the cyclical *changes* by creating a steady state. But even within that category some are better than others. RCOG specifically notes that "Newer generation COCs (Zoely, Yaz, Diane) are more effective than the older COCs". One woman claimed switching from Yasmine to Yaz made all the difference for her. Only difference is Yaz has 33% less ethinyl estradiol. Yaz is also the only birth control of any kind that is approved by the FDA for PMDD. Others, of course, may be used off label.

The estrogen in COCs is generally the same but different pills use different progestins. The single most popular progestin is levonorgestrel. Levonorgestrel is used in many COCs , ALL hormonal IUDs, and is the active ingredient in Plan B. Levonorgestrel is the worst progestin[10] for women with PMDD as it has many properties that exacerbate PMDD symptoms.

Yaz is generally recommended because it uses drospirenone as it's progestin and drospirenone has many properties that are of *benefit* to women with PMDD.

That said some women find COCs make their symptoms worse, or if they have migraine with aura they cannot take estrogen. Those women may find that Slynd, which is a POP, helps considerably. Slynd uniquely (among POPs) contains drospirenone which is the synthetic progestin found in Yaz. Drospirenone has anti-androgenic and anti-mineralocorticoid properties which means it can help reduce symptoms like bloating, acne, and *mood swings*.

SSRIs are also not one thing and the way they work for PMDD is completely different[11] to how they work for everything else. Doctors hear that PMDD causes anxiety/depression during luteal and SSRIs are used to treat anxiety/depression so they throw a daily therapeutic dose at you and it causes long term side effects during a months long trial that puts you off ever trying an SSRI again.

But for PMDD it's an extremely low dose (p.26) during luteal only. Some women even microdose[12] *as needed*. There are **no** long term side effects because you're not on it long term. And because it's intermittent dosing you can switch every cycle until you find the most effective one with the least short term side effects. Honestly I don't know why they don't just prescribe a sampler pack to start.

If you've **tried everything** and nothing helps I have just one question. Have you tried Acupuncture? TCM? TMS? Ketamine? Psilocybin? CBD? CGB? Nootropics? Pepcid? Biofeedback? DBT? Voodoo? Osteopathy? Cat rescue? Wim Hof? Weightlifting? Seed cycling? GABA? Trampoline? Lysine? High doses of vitamin C? Integrative Medicine? Low histamine diet? Passionflower? Iron? Psyllium husk? Going for a walk? Magneeeseeum?

---

10 https://www.reddit.com/r/PMDD/wiki/index/birth_control/
11 https://www.reddit.com/r/Psychiatry/comments/17ji14g
12 https://www.reddit.com/r/PMDD/comments/1i1x31u

Honestly I saw a post yesterday in which a woman was incensed that her doctor suggested going for a walk. Can you believe it? Yes. Absolutely. Doctors recommend going for a walk for all sorts of things *because it helps*. We should all go for a walk everyday. "Touch grass" as the kids say. Much better than stewing in your own juices. And while you're out there try to find some awe.

TL;DR: If you are posting to seek treatment recommendations or feedback please *be specific* about what you have tried so far.

Recommended treatment options are here (p.22).

Supplements women with PMDD have said helped are here (p.284).

Random success stories are here.[13]

> Otherwise-Guidance31
> This is an excellent post. The subtle and nuanced differences between each of the BC and SSRI options are usually not appreciated by most other than those who have trialled several before finding one that fits.
>
> Add to that the possibility that sometimes the first options might make symptoms worse. And that even effective meds might make things worse before they get better... Then any kind of medication hesitancy or fear of man-made drugs etc. And it seems likely that the majority of sufferers never find an effective or optimal treatment regime.
>
> And it's absolutely true that the only people who are really in a position to take the lead in this journey are the sufferers themselves or maybe a committed partner. It's unlikely that most healthcare professionals involved will go beyond trialling first line options and suggesting alternatives if patients keep returning, asking to try something else.
>
>
> Apart-Caramel5389
> You are an all star for sharing this. Thank you.

The original post on the sub.[14]

---

13 https://www.reddit.com/r/PMDDpartners/wiki/index/personalsuccess/
14 https://www.reddit.com/r/PMDDpartners/comments/1mlotw9

Selected Posts

Other posts that feel important and/or representative. I debated lightly editing the comments as some are not helpful or even relevant. But then that's representative too …

The first post in the list is breathtaking. We get one of these about every six months. Each time I'm impressed by how measured the partners response is. As a mod I expect I'll have to delete a bunch of cussing – but the partners have long practice being polite in the face of unreason.

You can't do it for her and you can't do it alone.

PMDD doesn't have triggers, only excuses.

She's mad, you're there, that's it.

Greyrocking is a survival strategy, not a lifestyle choice.

The couples that make it are the ones that can work together against the common enemy.

Question

Sorry-Story4498 - November 9, 2024

How many of you actually support your partners during hell week?

Like how many of you actually take into consideration what she is going through and actively try to make her life easier?

I see multiple post about how her behavior affects you as the partner, but hardly if any posts about what you are doing to support her.

Most on here track their partners cycles, to know when hell week starts, and to mentally prepare for the worst.. but, and i know this might be an unpopular opinion…how about running a bath for her, get her favourite snacks, give her a care basket, give her a massage, buy flowers, etc? If you can track her cycle to mentally prepare for the worst surely that can be done do support her too?

I am by no means saying accept abusive behaviour, but I have found that support and comfort during hell week, works far better than just leaving her to her own demise.

> nogeologyhere
> When you receive hellish amounts of grief when doing your best to be supportive, and continued abuse if you get anything wrong, then eventually compassion fatigue sets in and it's hard to maintain. I think many people try very very hard for a very very long time, but eventually crack and struggle.
>
> > Sorry-Story4498 OP
> > How well do you deal with criticism in general? Do you practice active listening when she speaks about the things that you do wrong, or do you get defensive and then emotionally shut down?
> >
> > > Deviator_Stress
> > > I've just read through your various comments and I'm finding an accusatory tone in most of them
> > >
> > > You're commenting in a sub where people have come for support because they have been, and in many cases still are being, abused. And a big part of that abuse is the partner with PMDD heaping blame on them like you're doing right now. The truth is that when someone is having an episode their partner can't win. There is

literally nothing they can do to stop the episode. It doesn't matter how much they do around the house, how supportive they are, how emotionally tolerant they are - the abuse continues and it is soul destroying.

Out of interest, are you a person with PMDD who has found out their partner is on this sub and decided to make a new account to come and throw some blame around? Because that's what it feels like

vanthrowaway2160
JFC. The partners here can probably relate to one of the many instances where I've been screamed at for being a "lazy asshole" while doing the dishes after having made dinner after working my job after getting the kids ready after making breakfast for the 7th day in a row.

What brings us here goes way way beyond criticism.

runemforit
I would take on a lot of emotional and domestic labor, completely changed my domestic routines, and truly bent over backwards to accommodate her needs. I loved her. Still do. But when all those things became expectations, even outside of luteal, and the demands kept growing and the criticisms kept growing, I knew there was nothing I could do to make that relationship work for me. At some point, it's on her to recognize im a dumping ground and manage herself better.

There's a wide spectrum of severity and how well women manage this illness and how it affects their partners. Im glad you're posting something about holding us accountable. Its an important part of the conversation. But this is a supportive community, and many of us are dealing with domestic abuse from our baby mommas. Maybe it's OK that people have a place to vent that doesn't center around their partner's needs?

For the record, I completely jive with what you're saying.. but asking people who are putting up with verbal and physical abuse so they don't lose access to seeing their children whether they're drawing baths doesn't seem like it's in good faith to this community.

Edit: for the record, I truly did everything you're describing. the massages, the flowers, everything. The important question i had to ask myself is "what am I getting out of this?" and as much as it hurts, I made the right choice leaving.

Sorry-Story4498 OP
Your experience is totaly valid and i am so sorry that you needed to go through the hardships of supporting a partner with so many needs.

Clearly my question wasnt meant for you, however, I am sure you don't speak for the whole sub.

Thank you for your input.

> SchaubbinKnob
> They speak for anyone who is dealing with someone else's mental illness.
>
> We do our best as partners.
>
> We come here for support because we're exhausted.
>
> The question that matters is…
>
> Are you following a routine of health?!
>
> Therapy Exercise Diet
>
> Many people are on their own.
>
> Those lucky enough to have someone to lean on should be grateful. They should show their appreciation by working diligently and proactively to mitigate their circumstances.
>
> I never blame a cripple for needing a push uphill. However if they attack me while I'm doing it, I have a real issue.
>
> > Sorry-Story4498 OP
> > Your experience is totaly valid and i am so sorry that you needed to go through the hardships of supporting a partner with so many needs.
> >
> > Clearly my question wasnt meant for you, however, I am sure you don't speak for the whole sub.
> >
> > Thank you for your input.

Socalwarrior485
I don't anymore. It makes no difference before, during or after. Dysphoria is a hell of a drug.

Sorry-Story4498 OP
Im so sorry that you are going through such horrible times.

Socalwarrior485
The sad part is that it really doesn't affect me anymore, just her. The kids are grown.

I have absolutely no control over anyone's happiness except my own. She owns hers, and I've discovered that while I'm an amazing husband, the reality she creates in her mind is the only one that exists for her.

Again, nothing a partner does can make a person happy.

Sorry-Story4498 OP
Define happiness? How long has your partner suffered with pmdd, was she ever formally diagnosed?

Socalwarrior485
Yes, she was diagnosed about a year after we were married about 22 years ago. She tried treating it, but she has a hard time remembering to take pills (that's how we ended up with our first). After a couple tries that had side effects, she gave up and has now convinced herself that all of the problems are caused by others.

I define happiness as the absence of unhappiness. Seems circular, but it works for me. My life is super satisfying now. Things have been getting better so much. So, I'm happy. No matter how much she gets of anything, she repeats the cycle every month, and now with menopause coming, it's just drawn out.

She has a pretty good life. She's been a stay at home wife for 21+ years now. I do my share of domestic caring and also all of the home and auto repairs. My life is awesome. My older kids are at great universities and our youngest is 14 and a good kid. If she can't see how great her life is, there is nothing I can do.

> I've told her to stay off social media, but that's what she does
> with most of her time. Comparison is the thief of happiness.

dutchvonrabbit
Doesn't work or help. There is always a reason, to hone in and attack you.

Really doesn't matter how kind or considerate your are. I still do it for her because I love her and that's who I am. But there is always a reason.

> Sorry-Story4498 OP
> You sound like a wonderful partner, i am so sorry you need to go
> through such terrible times.
>
> Clearly my question wasn't meant for you.
>
> Thank you for your input.

Phew-ThatWasClose
This question shows a really deep lack of understanding and empathy. I don't know your history because you have none. If you've been lurking since February 2023 I would expect you to be a lot better informed. It's true that some women with PMDD have shitty partners. Those partners are not here.

We get two types of partners here. One is the earnest fellow with puppy dog eyes who just found out how the love of his life has this disorder and he googled "my partner has pmdd" and google sent him here. Those of us who are still bitter and reactive from our own damage tell that fellow to "Run!". The rest of us point to open communication, asking her what she needs, making a plan (p.58). looking at treatment (p.22), looking at supplements (p.284), changing diet and exercise habits, and generally working together to manage what is a chronic medical condition.

PMDD is a mixed bag. Diagnostic criteria (p.268) are any five of a possible eleven symptoms. Most women with PMDD do not experience rage as a symptom. For the earnest fellow who really just wants to know how to help his partner through a rough patch every cycle our advice helps, he and his partner manage the condition and live happily ever after. Or he leaves her. Either way he doesn't stick around here.

The rest of us do stick around because we have ongoing issues and need ongoing support, or we empathize and want to offer that support, or both. Often we are partners of women who do experience rage as a symptom and the disorder was undiagnosed and/or untreated for years, sometimes decades.

Imagine what that is like. Being verbally assaulted for 7-10 days seemingly at random. What was fine yesterday is suddenly the worst sin imaginable. Whatever the worst sin imaginable was last time is now unimportant. Try as you might to do as she asks you're wrong, and you should have known, and how could you even, and why haven't you done this yet, and DON'T TELL ME TO CALM DOWN, and pay attention when I talk to you, and DON'T YOU DARE WALK AWAY!

You bet your sweet bippy we tried everything. And many of us lost ourselves in the process. The post immediately below this one is from a guy who doesn't know who he is anymore and is so beaten down he can't even recognize there is an exit much less use it. Most of us have been there. Some of us are there right now. Drowning in a sea of abuse clinging to "But I love her." when there is none coming the other direction and our cup has been so so empty for so so long.

But sure. Maybe active listening will help.

> **Sorry-Story4498 OP**
> Thank you for your thesis. Im glad you got that off your chest. Clearly my question wasn't meant for you, and surely you dont speak for everyone on this sub.

>> **Phew-ThatWasClose**
>> You asked how many have tried just supporting their partner through luteal. Then every time someone says "I did." or "I still do" you claim your question wasn't for them. So who is your question for? What are you after?

>> **theatergeek1**
>> Seems like your question isn't for anyone here or you are looking for a kind of contrite answer or hope that those kind of table stakes will have a meaningful impact on the cold hostility or rage or irrational thought salads or paranoia that we have all experienced during luteal. It's worse when she isn't exercising or taking her meds or leaning on therapist or anyone else. Flowers only help IF she is also doing every damn thing to be a loving partner to US by actively managing the beast that is PMDD

Phew-ThatWasClose_
Ngl, "thought salad" made me laugh. That's the perfect description. :)

its_FORTY
To be honest, the passive aggressive manner in which you've responded to everyone who has takent the time to reply to you looks a LOT like the irrational behavior most of us are living through during PMDD luteal phases. What's up with that?

_d_o_o_d__
Well said, brother!

PieceKind2819
I feel that most of the partners in the sub are further down the hypothetical timeline with their pwPMDD.

Most partners have a specific archetype for being "saviors", and at the very least have the awareness and empathy to try and improve the situation overall.

Many come here being solution focused and are in search of more profound tools beyond the standard spousal support frameworks, processes, systems, hired help (nannies, housecleaners, assistants, etc) that most of us have attempted to implement in the past.

If it were that easy, I can guarantee most of us would have been giddy to find a solution and we definitely wouldn't find ourselves posting on this sub.

If fact, most of us are in this situation due to trying to help too much and ultimately lost ourselves in the process.

Sorry-Story4498 OP
You surely can't speak for everyone's experience on this sub, or do you identify as most people? In which case, i am really sorry that you have gone through so much due to pmdd.

Another highly unpopular opinion, some partners lack relationship experience, emotional maturity or common sense and havent tried or even thought of the things i mention in my post.

Thank you for your input.

> PieceKind2819
> Do you have PMDD? Are you aware of how it functions? Are you aware of the underlying causes?
>
> There is a very clear archetype of person who has PMDD. Unfortunately, this archetype has the traits you mentioned (lack of emotional maturity, common sense, proper relationship modeling, etc). This is more than likely due to the environment and familial dynamics that caused the PMDD. There is a reason that over 85% of sufferers of PMDD also have a history of trauma or CPTSD.
>
> This is not an issue with abnormal hormone function, this is an issue with normal hormone function and how it relates to an abnormal emotional response system.
>
> The reason all of our situations are similar is because all of our partners have varying degrees of trauma, and with this includes varying degrees of symptom overlap (BPD, NPD, CPTSD, ADHD, ASD).
>
> The root cause in all of the labels mentioned is CPTSD and/or trauma.

> vanthrowaway2160
> Raises hand to join in with PieceKind2819.
>
> "Do you think just because you did (one of a huge list of tasks that you do) that makes everything better?"

PieceKind2819
I also would add that half of the sufferers experience cyclical bouts of dismissive avoidant behavior and they ramp up the distancing strategies.

In my experience, the last thing my ex-partner wanted me to do was to "lean in". When I did attempt to do any of these things I was baited into an argument, followed by being blocked on all devices and not spoken to for several weeks as a form of punishment and control.

There is literally a post within the last day of another person being blocked on all devices for no apparent reason.

I am more than happy to breakdown the psychological underpinnings of the fight, flight, and freeze response.

The partner isn't the source of the trauma, the partner is the intimacy trigger to the trauma. We are the match and the trauma is the gasoline. It's up to the sufferer to heal the gasoline, as it was more than likely experienced long before the relationship came into existence.

__d_o_o_d__
When you go that route what happens is the flowers you got are wrong, the treat you got was too small or too few, the chores you did are now solely your responsibility in perpetuity, the nice card you left for her gets twisted into an insult. The best thing you can do is get out of the danger zone while the battle is on

> its_FORTY
> Yep..
>
> You: "Hey honey, I got you some fresh flowers on the way home from work - I love you!"
>
> Her: "These aren't even the type of flowers I like, you should know that by now. Did you buy the wrong flowers just to hurt me? Why would you do that to me? Are you trying to hide something by distracting me with flowers? I know you're having an affair, why don't you just divorce me already. I know you want to."

AcadiaPrimary614
I don't do much anymore, everything I've tried in the past either resulted in being snapped at or being refused.

After over ten years of trying everything I made the decision that we should have separate bedrooms and go low/no contact for the bad times (which is almost always now thanks to her being in perimenopause).

I'm sick of the conflict and having my soul slowly crushed but I'm hoping this will see us through to when she levels out or the kids are all 18.

Quote_Sure

Support and comfort when they actually want it yes. But often times, my offers of support and comfort are rejected. Which is absolutely fine if that's what she wants, until she turns it around later and tries to accuse me of being neglectful. Or tries to go through a character assassination. Or accuses me of not being a man and apparently there are other men out there that would be better. Even though I put my partner first before everything.

I think most of us here absolutely want to support our partners, but when things get spicy and you get used as a verbal punch bag, that's when you get the posts that you are describing. About how the behaviour affects us, and this group should be a safe space for us to express ourselves when there isn't anywhere else.

SilhouetteEvelyn
I think there's nothing wrong with the others focusing on how they can distance themselves during the hell week, especially considering how some can be worse than others.

I personally do a mix of both. I still want her to feel like I'm here despite everything she's going through, so I just order a bouquet from Bouqs, and have it delivered straight to her. She blocks me sometimes for no reason at all, so I make sure to inform her sister in advance.

When she reaches out, I try not to bring up anything else. I just welcome her, talk to her about whatever she wants to talk to.

CheckZealousideal493
I was supportive for a year. But it then becomes a case of self care is not selfish. One can't take so much shite and it not begin to affect them. Some folk, no matter how beautiful they are when not in as you say 'hell week'.. doesn't outweigh the burden and drain during 'hell week'. Relationship is a choice and life is too short to be with someone who can not be themselves

The original post on the sub.[1]

"The one below this one"[2] has since been deleted.

It's in the archive[3] if you really want to see it.

---

1   https://www.reddit.com/r/PMDDpartners/comments/1gnb071
2   https://www.reddit.com/r/PMDDpartners/comments/1gmojkd
3   https://arctic-shift.photon-reddit.com/search?fun=ids&ids=t3_1gmojkd

What if the luteal talk is honest?

theSeaOfAsh December 31, 2024

This time around, my wife with PMDD (and probably other personality disorders) had told me several hurtful things that go straight to the very base of our relationship. Now I'm wondering if I should do as she does, which is to say there's a grain of truth to whatever venom comes out in these hormonal explosions. Shouldn't I just accept that she thought I'm evil the very first time we met and I am a horrible person to her most of the time and she actively doesn't want to care about what I want in life, etc. Shouldn't I just get serious about separating when there's nothing good left that she hasn't broken?

P.S. I'm not even sure it's pmdd anymore, because there are no "good days" after or before luteal anymore. There was at least one hugely problematic day every week in the last couple of months.

> pdvdw
> In my experience, it seems to compound if the other person isn't taking accountability for the horrible things they said while in the midst of it. Now they dig in their heels and start believing the things they said instead of taking accountability. Then it bleeds into every day life.
>
> The only solution in my mind to dealing with PMDD is accountability. If they refuse then there's trouble.
>
> Source: in the same situation as you right now
>
>> Less_Rich844
>> That's how it's been with my wife. No accountability. It makes it hurt so much worse
>
>> The90sWereYesterday
>> You are not alone. I have been lying in bed awake for three hours staring at the ceiling and asking myself the same question. My wife just hit follicular and has shifted back into super lovey mode, so I am trying to breathe and let my guard down for a few weeks of normalcy. We've been on this ride for decades, but we only received the PMDD diagnosis a few months ago. So, I find myself wrestling with which version of my wife I should believe and listen to. I also struggle with the nagging feeling that there is truth in the words and feelings expressed during luteal.

If you read the posts in r/PMDD[4] you will find lots of women proudly proclaiming that luteal gives them clarity and connects their true feelings. Those posts are often paired with the celebration that they quit their jobs or ended their relationships because they could see that those things were the problem. Every time I see that, I wonder and worry if luteal feelings are prevalent outside of hell week. I also wonder if those women were really in bad situations, or if their altered PMDD reality is leading them to make self-destructive choices. My wife swears that the luteal outbursts aren't real feelings, but it is hard to believe that. My wife will tell me that she doesn't even remember saying some of the most hurtful and cutting things that have been said in luteal. Which makes me not know what to believe. My therapist also likes to remind me that every woman is different, and every woman's PMDD symptoms and responses are different; so, that doesn't help answer any questions either. So, I think I've landed on the conclusion that we don't really know, and they may not really know either.

Sadly, we don't know much about PMDD. Nobody seems to. It isn't well studied and there aren't clear solutions and treatments that will work for everyone. This makes it hard for everyone affected by this. You are not alone, but your situation is also unique to you and your wife. My wife was prescribed medicine which seems to be helping, so I am optimistic.

We are both in individual therapy, which I hope helps too. My therapist is great for reminding me that I'm not crazy, and the rage and vitriol spewed are not ok and not my fault. She has also been helpful in understanding PMDD and perimenopause symptoms. I don't know how old you are, but this gets much worse with perimenopause. If your wife is 40+, this is a significant factor.

My advice, get some help if you haven't already. Starting with getting your wife help to treat the PMDD. Talk to her a few days after her period ends, that seems to be the safest time that I find to talk with my wife. Tell her that you are concerned for her and for the relationship. Ask her to please seek treatment, or to try something different if she already being treated. Get yourself to therapy if you haven't already. Once things are better regulated, then maybe you and wife should talk about your feelings and evaluate how you both really feel. These conversations and decisions shouldn't happen during the luteal phase. Then you can maybe have a conversation and try to discover what real, rational feelings exist.

That being said, my advice is based only on what I have experienced. I don't think anyone outside of this forum really understands what PMDD partners experience. Until I found this subreddit I didn't think anyone

---

4   https://www.reddit.com/r/PMDD/

would even believe me if I told them what my life was like.

Every situation and experience is unique, so you have to decide for you. If you still love your wife and can still see the person you fell in love with shining through from time to time, then it may be worth working through it. It is you and her against the PMDD. Perhaps in time you can get a clearer understanding of what weight, if any, the things said in luteal have. Good luck.

> SantoriniBisque
> Get out of the relationship

>> The90sWereYesterday
>> Is that for me, or OP? Either way, that recommendation in a vacuum is a hollow sentiment. I'm sorry for whatever your experience has been, but sometimes relationships are complicated. Ending a marriage is not always as simple as just getting out of the relationship. PMDD sort of falls under the, "through sickness and health" realm.

>>> Mart243
>>> "through sickness" doesn't mean abuse. I don't know of the words your wife said can be considered abuse, or just more of a helpless cry for help

Mart243
Once perimenopause hits things seem to go out of control. I could "handle" the pmdd cycles, and did for 6 years (after a 20 years relationship with someone that had borderline personality disorder) but it seems like perimenopause was draining her more (much less good days) so she ended up putting the relationship on "pause" to have some space to think since she could not see a future. I think that she is of the disorganized attachment type which is amplified by pmdd. She also started HRT which likely messed things up further since it takes a while to settle, if it settles..

She did say quite a few times lately that PMDD was simply removing the veil of what she was truly feeling.. sadly, with disorganized attachment your feelings are all over the place. Add some childhood trauma in there which commonly resurfaces at perimenopause and things get interesting... So yeah, not super positive outlook but the only thing I can do it take care of myself in the meantime

Total_Plankton_3830 January 9, 2025
I have PMDD and so does my partner. I was diagnosed years ago and she only recently but we both have struggled for a decade.

From my experience- PMDD only tells me lies. It amplifies things that already feel like shit, and plants lies about other things.

In my window I am totally unable to access the logical parts of my brain. I am totally hi jacked and can only draw negative conclusions and outcomes.

On a good day out of luteal this is not the case. My brain literally does not seem to have access to my full spectrum of tools, emotions and thinking processes when I am in my window.

The most valuable tool that I have gathered when in this space came from my therapist. She also has PMDD and has explained that when I find myself here and feel like doing something extreme- the only thing to do is NOTHING. Until it blows over. To avoid burning down my life and relationships.

My partner is trying to learn this but struggles heavily. She lets the rage take her over. She burns down relationships (our relationship even) and is super self destructive. She feels deep shame when this happens which increases the rage that she feels. She runs from accountability literally ending and avoiding any relationship that might hold her accountable.

And then she gets out of luteal and love bombs (still not taking much accountability but giving bare minimum apologies or acknowledgement without any commitment to real repair) and acts like it never happened. Until next month. Or actually 2 weeks.

I have PMDD so I am capable of extending grace. But this is hard when she takes no accountability. Extending grace to a person who won't take any accountability for the harm they cause feels more like enabling their behavior.

> The90sWereYesterday
> Thank you for this. This is a valuable perspective since you experience it on both sides of the PMDD coin. The lack of accountability is, and has been, disheartening for me. I'm working on the giving grace part now that we can connect some of it to PMDD, but it can be hard. All of this is difficult. Thank you again for responding.

Phew-ThatWasClose
Some women with PMDD, and even some partners, will say luteal just
brings out the valid points she would normally just let pass. So we
shouldn't ignore what's said in luteal. We should listen and validate and
respect. And I disagree. PMDD lies, Always. It's all lies.

There is no kernal of truth that only the dysphoria of PMDD can bring to
the surface. PMDD doesn't somehow grant women second sight and
wisdom beyond Solomon's dreams. There's no "respectful" position being
voiced. It's nonsense, garbage, crap, bullshit. She's angry, you're there.
That's it.

The only "kernal of truth" is that You are sometimes annoying. That is true
of everyone, everywhere, throughout all of time. That's not a "kernal of
truth". That's not some deep hidden knowledge that is only revealed by
the psychotic rage of luteal. That is background noise.

Background noise that PMDD seizes on, magnifies, amplifies, and
sharpens in an effort to eviscerate you. Don't fall for it. It's lies, hokum,
fluff, trash, malarkey.

OTOH - If she says "Can you do the dishes tonight?" and you say "What?
Are you in luteal or something?" then you're a jerk. It's all context.

> Less_Rich844
> I needed to hear this today. Thank you.

SantoriniBisque
It's a dead end and you will never come out happy. Just leave the
relationship. You'll feel better in several months after questioning yourself
if you did the right choice or feeling the regret. It is normal and stay
strong.

She won't change and you are probably right it is possible not PMDD or
only PMDD. My experience she appears to have other PDs. Or
combination. Hard to label when she is in a spectrum of wide range of
disorder.

Sammovt
I had a similar experience with my longtime now ex-girlfriend who tried to
blame all of her fucked up behavior on being "autistic." Here is a link to
my post about that if anybody is interested. In my experience, if you are

seriously questioning whether you should be getting out of your relationship, it is already past the time that you should have gotten out.

If it walks like a duck and talks like a duck, it's probably a duck. https://www.reddit.com/r/autism/s/LUgaDEGwbv[5]

grizzard619
So, my wife (35) and I had a difficult last couple of years. I'm talking huge, completely irrational blow ups every week. And it continued like that for over a year. There were also other behavior changes that I will not get into, but suffice to say, we were ready to sign papers and go our separate ways. The biggest thing that changed/catalyst was her psychiatric nurse practitioner putting her on Abilify (apriprazole) which, in low doses, is used to treat "irritability associated with autism". It took about three months to fully take affect, but I got my best friend back.

In regard to the luteal talk being honest, I'll just add "a broken clock is right twice a day".

Edit to add: She still has her bad days during luteal, but it is FAR, FAR more manageable than before.

Specific-Rest1631
This is not meant to be disparaging in any way to women, but you have to understand that when she is talking to you she is telling you what her reality is right now. Not 5 years ago, or 5 years from now, not even 5 minutes from now. That doesn't mean it isn't true, but it's rarely true the way we think of it. The best thing you can do for yourself other than leave is to do work on developing your ego. The stronger your ego is the more resilient you will be to anyone telling you who or what you are.

Edit, just to tell you this thought has run through my mind many times in the last 10 years, and at one point I let it really grind me down and destroy my sense of self.

Baking_Dude February1, 2025
This is my fear. These are my thoughts over the past 18 years. The words she said to me, using my past against me, hurtful, cruel, mean, insulting, denigrating…she says "making you feel bad makes my pain less" yet "it's not me saying those words". But they're words and thoughts within her…so how can they not be part of her? I cannot wrap my head

---

5   http://www.reddit.com/r/autism/s/LUgaDEGwbv

around the distancing from her words and actions, her absolution from wrongdoing because she has pmdd.

The original post on the sub.[6]

---

6   https://www.reddit.com/r/PMDDpartners/comments/1hqbmln

Psychedelics

dontwakethellama March 7, 2024

So, the purpose of this post is going to be purely informational in regards to YOU, the PARTNER, using psychedelics and how it can have a change of perspective that actually helps you with PMDD and a lot of other things in your life. If you are anti-psychedelic, that's cool... You can possibly still take something away from reading this. I don't smoke or drink or do anything... I was a DARE kid. I still don't like pot or alcohol and have been anti-drug for all my life.... Psychedelics are the only things I feel pretty positive about because I think they can actually have a benefit.

In a few of my previous comments, some of you may have seen that I had a huge change in my perspective of PMDD after taking psychedelic mushrooms (I purge my history every so often, so I don't believe they're still there). This is a quick breakdown of why I think it was one of the most impactful things I've done for my life and my relationship(s).
I have only taken mushrooms a few times in my life (I'm nearly 40). Most of them were medium doses that had really cool visuals and made me think in funny different ways that were pretty cool.

ONE time, my mind went to a different universe. (This is long and will seem like it goes off the rails a bit, but I promise I'll bring it back at the end.)

During that trip, I was convinced that all of us and every living thing in the universe are connected by energy and that we're all reporting our experiences through that energy back to a centralized consciousness. Think about how our nerve endings are reporting back to our brain... Kinda like that. Everything became clear in that moment. I was a part of this centralized consciousness and, therefore, was a creator of everything. The multiple/infinite universe theories became completely understandable because I knew that I could think up ANYTHING and create that reality... boom, that's another universe created. The alternate and infinite possibilities of universes don't necessarily already exist, but they could with the immediacy of this centralized consciousness just thinking about it.

So then I started getting really sad/upset. If I AM this centralized consciousness and I'm creating everything and everyone, then everything and everyone is only a figment of my imagination. Poof... I realized that all time is existing in a single point, not a line like we think... Any memories that I have are actually me just thinking of them RIGHT NOW and they never actually existed before that moment. So I started crying because my Mom, Dad, wife, friends never actually existed. I created them in my imagination... I'm only remembering memories that I'm actually creating at that exact moment.

Then, I realized that time is infinite and, as the creator, I will be living this imagined reality for eternity. I wanted out… Why would I continue living a life where I have to go to a job that I hate… Why do I have to deal with crappy people? Why the heck did I create all these weird things? Why did I design physics in such a way that I can't fly around and have fun?

The only way out of this is death… I started thinking that people who commit suicide may actually be enlightened and moving on to create different realities for themselves. I thought about suicide for myself so I could go create something new. I cried and told my wife "I'm really going to miss you… You were one of my favorite creations". She was understandably worried about that kind of talk and stuck with me until I started coming down. I stopped wanting to commit suicide and figured that I had enough enjoyment from this world to go ahead and stay until I die of old age… But I wasn't going to continue living a life with parts that suck. No more crappy jobs and no time for crappy people. I started planning how to run away and escape to a tropical place where my current retirement balance could let us live like royalty until we die. That mindset actually lasted for about a week where I was confused about what was real and thought there was still a possibility that I AM a part of this centralized intelligence and that all energy is connected.

So, what the heck does this have to do with PMDD? During that entire trip and the following week, I was CONVINCED that it was all real. Alcohol makes you do and think things that you wouldn't normally do, but you know you're drunk and alcohol is the reason. Pot is similar… You feel the difference and enjoy the experience of pot, knowing that it's pot the whole time. With mushrooms, the line of reality got blurred. I no longer believed that mushrooms were causing this trip… I believed that they were a key that opened up my ability to see the ACTUAL reality.

After getting myself back to reality and understanding it was a mushroom trip, I'm able to see that my wife can have a completely different sense of reality during her "PMDD trip". I understand first-hand that there is a chemical reaction that can affect the brain and shift the reality for that individual… And it's not controllable… It cannot be reasoned with.

I use that understanding to give her grace during any rage or outburst at me or anyone else during the PMDD time. I understand that this is not actually her, and I'll get to be with the real her when she "comes down" again. I support her through coming back to reality and let her know that she doesn't have to be ashamed or feel guilty because I KNOW that wasn't her talking.

If any of you have taken mushrooms (or maybe LSD or DMT or Ketamine… I haven't tried them), then you may know what I'm talking about if you've crossed that dosage level.

Anyway, thanks for reading again. I'm sorry my posts are so long… I'm not great at being concise and feeling like I still get the same impact.

TLDR: Psychedelic mushrooms made me think I was in a different reality and I couldn't be reasoned with or convinced otherwise. After they wore off, I gained a permanent new understanding that my wife is experiencing a different reality during PMDD episodes, so I am able to give her grace.

> Mcfly-1983
> Dude, that resonates. I'm going to sit with that insight, thank you for sharing.
>
> seeyouspace__cowboy
> As someone with PMDD I think psychedelics are great for getting in touch with your emotions when PMDD symptoms start acting up. I recently got off birth control which was great for managing my pmdd. Unfortunately I had to get off it for unrelated reasons but in no time I was back to where I was with PMDD, severely anxious about every part of my life (especially my relationship) , severely depressed , and feeling like I wanted to self harm again . My symptoms get more intense a few days prior to my period and I just couldn't handle my anxiety anymore . Instead of imploding my life I remembered I had a mushroom microdose pill from a while ago . That shut my anxiety right up . I was able to be much more present and better articulate what I was feeling . Shrooms also make me more emotional so I had a good cry too because for whatever reason I haven't been able to cry lately . PMDD feels like holding a monster in a cage . I'm still trying to figure what's good to do during that time period and experimenting on microdosing with shrooms and marijuana during that time . I think shrooms are great because it's so easy to not realize what's real or not during that time it's hard to explain. I feel like shrooms gives me a better understanding of where the anxiety comes from as well as being great when you need to just let emotions out .

The original post on the sub.[7]

---

7   https://www.reddit.com/r/PMDDpartners/comments/1b90dao

PMDD reality

Redskrot – October 23, 2024

Hi, my wife has had PMDD for about 9 years.

She is in mid luteal right now and last night i slipped and was unable to avoid a rage outburst. It wasnt a big one, so no real worry but it got me thinking.

Often during these rages she accuses me of a lot of things. Things i have done, said or even thought. Most of these things has never happened. Even really easy things to check from during the same day she "lie" about and no argument can make her change her mind.

I always thought that she knows all too well that the accusations are lies but she uses it to fuel her rage and it makes her feel a bit better to have a reason to be angry.

So my question is; does she know she is lying? Or does she really believe these things? If she does, then in some sense i really am the asshole, and it must be really strange for her that i am defending my self?

Edit:

This thread just started as a shower thought. However, the comments has been beyond great and this turned out to be extremely educational for at least me. I am sorry if I'm not responding to everyone, but be assure i greatly value all the input.

Phew-ThatWasClose
She's not lying to you. She's a total sweetheart and would never do that. The PMDD, on the other hand, lies like an orange rapist with dementia.

As you noted there's no argument can make her change her mind. So don't argue. The more you argue the more she digs in her heels and the more real it becomes. Just being there gives her a target she can yell at and the lie becomes more real with each repetition. Sometimes greyrocking is necessary, but it is always better to walk away if you can. A half hour to calm down is the number one doctor recommended way to deal with anger.

Do talk about it next week, during follicular, to make sure she knows it's not true. Otherwise it becomes part of the tapestry and your good name degrades over time.

EtoileNoirr
May I ask what is grey rocking?

> Phew-ThatWasClose
> Greyrocking is a survival tactic sometimes used by victims of abuse. Is similar to being attacked by a bear. You make yourself as uninteresting as possible, like a grey rock, and the bear may not kill you and eat you. With verbal abuse it means you don't respond, no matter what, in the hope your abuser will get bored and go away. It doesn't work very well, but responding in any way will escalate things so greyrocking is often the least bad option.
>
> Much better to walk away, but that's not always possible.

>> OsakaWilson
>> "Much better to walk away, but that's not always possible."
>>
>> She goes after me when I am driving and cannot simply get away. I've walked out into a snow storm to get away in the past.

>>> Phew-ThatWasClose
>>> I've had her jump in the car when I was trying to escape and in my desperation I had the brilliant idea the I would drive to the police station. After about a block I realized there was no way I could drive 2 miles through traffic with her yelling at me so I turned around, parked it back where it was, and fled on foot. She followed for eight blocks in her bare feet.
>>>
>>> That story is why the sample plan (p.69) is explicit about only using the car when it is safe to do so. :(
>>>
>>> If you're actually driving when it begins ... that's not safe. Once it took me 2 hours to make the half hour drive home when I picked her up from *the psych ward* because I had to pull over and take breaks. We still have the busted windshield in the van. We told the kids it was a rock kicked up by a truck.
>>>
>>> Yeah, not always possible but so so so much better if you can.

>>>> Catgirl_78
>>>> Wow. This is really not acceptable behavior in any way. What treatments is she using for her PMDD? How proactive is she in getting help for this condition? It should be her number one priority. I'm so sorry you're dealing with such a difficult

situation. I have severe pmdd, but mine is more directed inward. I isolate, stay in bed, get super depressed and sometimes suicidal. I never take it out on other people. It's a terrible disease, but having it does not excuse the abuse she is inflicting on you.

Phew-ThatWasClose
Thanks for your concern. Both those incidents happened during peri. Eventually she got on a mood stabilizer (lamictol) and started DBT. Things improved 1000x almost overnight. She's in menopause now so no more PMDD. Still one day at a time but making progress.

Catgirl_78

Infoseek456
So once menopause actually hits- the PMDD does really go away?

I'm getting close to that finish line, and the thought there is an end in sight has really been one of the few things to keep me going.

I've heard/read mixed things, that post-menopause brings its own brand of chemical imbalances and the saga continues.

I fear we'll never make it once the kids are fully grown and gone if this doesn't go away...

Phew-ThatWasClose
No cycle = No cycle related disorder.

No menstruation = No *pre*-menstruation.

Not to say there may not be other medical issues, but both RCOG and ACOG list chemical menopause and surgical menopause as last resort treatment for extreme cases. Natural menopause, obviously, being preferred.

If your lovely partner is in peri make sure to check out what DT has posted[8] about it.

EitherAccountant6736
I'm curious what happens to all of the trauma that was the root cause in the first place.

All of those patterns can't realistically just disappear into thin air.

> Infoseek456
> She'll still have all the underlying issues, just not the PMDD exacerbation of them. How she behaves on a "regular" day will become par for the course.
>
> So, we can just be jerks "regular style" ?.

redskrot OP
Thanks, very good points.
We have trouble talking about it even during follicular. She gets really grumpy if i raise it and walk away. And she absolutely won't talk with a professional. I am also a bit afraid of ruining the good weeks.

Time-Place5719
I wonder when they start believing this as reality.

Baloneous_V
Protecting your own sanity and not slipping into being gaslit becomes your priority at some point... but playing on the edge of reality with her like you are now is how it starts.

Like phew said, it's a lot harder to rewrite history and take that tapestry down than it is to defend it in real time, every time (by not interacting with it). No need to argue.

You become stronger and more anchored to reality with consistent responses to these events. I don't know yet if it ends up helping the dysphoric partner, but that's not the point after a certain stage. You're almost there I'd say.

---

8   https://www.reddit.com/r/PMDD/comments/1f46img/comment/lkow98r/

QuercusSambucus
My wife says that there are definitely psychotic elements to PMDD.
Especially if things like alcohol are involved. Perception is literally
disconnected from reality.

Quitchabitchin89
Long time lurker and first time responding. Grateful to have come
across this group and for all the helpful information to process and to
get through each month.

Yes and I have come to realize that for some people with PMDD, my
wife included, during the luteal period of the month, to cope with her
own demons, the release valve for her is a verbal garbage dump of all
her insecurities and anxiety for that month. The unlock was after I
realized to truly not take it personally, to greyrock and to try to make it
a game to distance myself mentally as a third party witness to see what
kind of rediculous things she can say. It is a little easier to cope with it.
She feels better after the release of pressure and we move on. But it is
not easy and we try to build our love back during the rest of the month.

HusbandofPMDD
Label it as abuse and ask if she's interested in recording these
interactions (with consent)

Temporary-County-356
I believe there is a spiritual element to PMDD as well.

Efficient-Pattern189
Explain please

Temporary-County-356
In many religions and parts of the world the spiritual world is very
real. The pmdd is something happening but the escalation is the
spirits coming out and causing destruction. Meaning the enemy isn't
playing fair but used the already fucked up person to add more fuel
to the fire and attach demons to the person. Just talk to some of
these women if they have experienced SA. That opens the door to
many spirits, not their fault but is the world we live in. It takes
incredible effort, prayer and belief in a higher power to change ways.
It also includes the humbling of one's self. Not many will do so. I
came to the conclusion once I realize that a woman's cycle is

already a vulnerable/sensitive time in a woman's life. I didn't say it was fair but look into the spiritual meaning of it. Many women with pmdd aren't living their life purpose, have trauma, and aren't living a healthy lifestyle. There is a spiritual aspect to this. Having constant negative thoughts is not normal. It's like they are being bombarded by external force all that negativity and they spit it out to everyone else. Causing havoc and broken relationships which is exactly what the powers that be want. A healthy and empowered woman is going to have to fight against the current and win she must the battle in her mind. This is a literal fight against life and death because suicide ideation and actual attempts is common with pmdd. This is literal spiritual warfare against women.

Far-Information-1127
how long until she accuses you of something very serious and then tells someone else?

iloveherbuticant
Oh...it has happened. I used to care. Now I can care much less what other people hear and believe. I know who I am and what I did or didn't do.

Justchristinen
I don't want to butt in where not wanted - I'm a 40yo f with pmdd and have been married 10 years. Ama. (I've done this before but always happy to answer more questions).

OP - let me know if you're interested in a pmdd opinion.

redskrot OP
Thank you for trying to help.

What i would really like to learn is how I should behave during luteal to optimizing the chances of keeping my wife happy and feeling ok.

Feel like whatever i do it fails. I do basically every chores, solely taking care of our three kids, cooking cleaning etc. All while walking a bit on eggshells to not annoy her.

If i do any mistakes she might explode. If she can't find anything wrong, she sometimes lay out traps. Like intentionally leaving her dishes at the table when I'm not seeing, and if i don't fix it during the evening she use that to attack me.

In rare occasions she can't find a reason to attack she might go into crying. She won't tell me what's wrong but if i don't console her in a perfect way she pounce.

When she attacks it's also really really hard to not go in defencive mode which makes it all worse.

All tips are welcome. I just want a happy and loving wife and are willing to do a lot to get that.

Phew-ThatWasClose
There is no "should". If the PMDD wants to fight the PMDD will find a way. As you have noted the PMDD is not above setting traps and if that doesn't work the PMDD will make shit up. You are wrong no matter what you do so you may as well just do what is right.

The couples that make it are the ones that work together against the common enemy. It sounds like you have gone way above and beyond to try and make this thing work. What is she doing?

Read this about vitamins and supplements (p.284).

Read this about treatments (p.22).

Read this about eggshells (p.54).

Read this about apologizing (p.117).

Read this about what others have to say (p.30).

You gotta have the tough conversation during follicular. You can't do it alone.

Carroto_
Hi, I'm the partner with PMDD.
I seriously thought you were my husband when I read the post…
Except we haven't had the bad episode in a while!

Some things that helped us during my extreme rage/accusing husband/or any anger: Create a pausing moment. Together.

When we come to an argument, one of us will reach out hand to hold hands. It's a sign for each other, "I still love you, I'm raging and I can't stop. I'm really angry-feeling. I don't know what to do myself either. I feel bad and angry at the same time."Usually all that feelings are combined in me when I'm raging. All this messages were built on overtime.

That said… this is still a team effort…Make sure to talk with her. Does she know what she's doing? Did she hear what you have to say? Did she feel like she's been heard?

Just something that's been working with us… Married and together for 11years. PMDD can be worked on and becomes less of an issue within the relationship through teamwork.

Justchristinen
So sorry you're in this cycle with her.

First, off I would say she has a massive responsibility to get help and do whatever she can to make this awful disorder affect those she loves less. That was always my driving factor at seeking treatment.

Second, how does she act around the kids?

Third, if anything regardless of reason is touching on abuse you need to make an exit plan. I think she needs to understand the seriousness of your pain and your responsibility to your family. I don't have kids but I grew ups with emotionally unstable parents and that's a whole other conversation.

There are effective treatments, and menopause does happen and will resolve the pmdd.

It sounds like she's weaponizing this condition instead of trying to overcome a bit. Is that harsh? Maybe. But so is knowing you have this condition and making everyone in your path your victim.

I went through huge phases of self harm and self loathing, suicidal ideation, psychosis, fatigue, insomnia, a bipolar diagnosis. I understand it's so hard but retreating into it isn't the answer.

Justchristinen
And about what you can do - set your boundaries firmly. Say you won't engage with certain things, and say you can listen if she needs to talk about how she feels but you can't accept all the

responsibility for it.
For annoying things - roommate stuff. My husband takes great care not to slam cupboards (he doesn't mean to he just closes things hard), takes the garbage out more often so there isn't weird smells, makes sure to rinse dish rags, room mate stuff lol

EitherAccountant6736
Honestly the question you just asked would be enabling her bad behavior.

During luteal her emotional response system is in overdrive (there's another guy on here who has the science mapped out in a book that he's working on).

The level of her reactions depends on if she is actively trying to combat the triggers, while also healing the underlying trauma that is causing the triggers.

It's not your responsibility to put emotional guard rails in place. What you can do is focus on how you react to the situations. Most of us reduce contact and focus on other aspects of life.

Maze187187
We can't tell you because everyone is different but in the case of my wife she beliefs these things in these moments and often repeats them many times. She often can't remember the details of the fights when she is normal again.

While greyrocking is a decent tactic I started some time ago to not let her get away with this stuff because once you repeat it again and again then it becomes reality (to her at least and she remembers them like this later on). I try to correct the (in my opinion) wrong phrases everytime she repeats them in a very calm and not agressive tone. That works pretty good for me. And I got sick of deeling with the "alternate realities".

redskrot OP
I have tried to correct her but it just becomes a back and forth like "that's not how thing is" responded by "that's exactly like it is" in a forever circle.

Maze187187
You won't get her to admit it - the trick is to correct her 1 or 2 times

but after that you just repeat the right phrase when talking about it while she repeats her version. This way you won't admit to her version being right but won't have a constant fight over it. (an example not so abstract would be like we had a fight were she would constantly repeat the wrong sequence/order things have been said/done that really turned the "blamegame"). I hope you get what I mean - english is not my first language.

rockrnger
No way of knowing. Both probably.

You just have to believe whichever one makes it better for you.

EitherAccountant6736
It's a trauma response due to toxic shame. Her brain believes a lot of the things in the moment.

I wouldn't even say she believes the ideas, it's more of how she's interpreted the events and how it is putting her in danger at some subconscious level.

No_Result4069
I'm 23F with PMDD, and in my experience, when I'm ruminating and over thinking, it is very very real. No question about it, he IS cheating, he DOES hate me, he DOES think I'm ugly. There is no reasoning with me, everything going on in my head is factual and if he says any different then he is lying. Then once I get my period I realize those things aren't true, it was just the hormones.

So yes, she could 100% believe the lies her brain is telling her, PMDD is an illness that distorts reality and they way your brain processes things. It's hell for you but it's even more of a hell for us. Because once we "sober up" from the hormones, we realize how delusional and irrational we were and we feel like monsters. It's a possession. She is literally not in there, only the PMDD is in there. Though she probably has moments of clarity here and there during luteal, but the majority of the luteal phase is full of depression and anger and self-hatred.

Though that does not excuse her behavior. Taking out frustrations on others is never okay, and I hope that maybe in her follicular phase you can try to talk to her about ways she can manage the anger. It might hurt her, but I think leaving the house or going to a different room when she's acting this way is what is best. Eventually she will understand that her anger calms down when the source of her anger is gone, i.e. you. Or discuss medication. Lexapro works great for me, I'm not taking it at the moment (for reasons) but when I was on it I was COMPLETELY different. I'm actually thinking about taking it again bc it made me feel so good. But I think antidepressants could really help her manage PMDD, it's really the only solution as there's no cure for this illness.

I hope things get better for you and your partner. Even though she can't control her emotions, everyone has some amount of control over their reactions. Please please please don't let her continue this emotional/verbal abuse. If you love her enough to stay with her through PMDD then I hope you love her enough to get her help. I wish I had someone who cared enough to ask questions about how to help me. You seem very patient and I ask that you please keep this patience. She really needs your support right now. But as I said, don't tolerate abuse. If you have to leave her then leave, but I think she can turn this around. There is hope for everyone.

Historical_Series543
I appreciate you sharing. Much of the help I've received in trying to understand this disorder has come directly from sufferers sharing their lived experience. However, I have noticed a tendency for sufferers to share similar sentiments to yours which usually amount to "remember, if you think it's hard for you, it's worse for her". I know everyone experiences PMDD with varying degrees of intensity and varying expressions but I have to disagree. Not with the content of the sentiment but the utterence itself. I know I'm not alone in saying this but my partner experiences some pretty extreme amnesia about her behavior in luteal. Whole arguments, hurtful words, gaslighting, traps -all of it- just a vague and hazy memory of an unpleasant dream. Once luteal is over she's back and full of life and energy and love. I, on the other hand, have spent the last two weeks shouldering our entire household while fending off arguments based on an imaginary version of myself and clearing her path of triggers, I do not get the luxury of hormone induced amnesia. I have a clear recollection of all of it and I'm tired, real tired. And the creature I've survived, who couldn't stand the sight of me, now wants love, affection, sex, help with projects and to never leave my proximity. By that time she's the last person I want to see let alone be intimate with. And so I'm faced with a choice, take the time and distance I need (which only after luteal can I afford to take) to recover, or pretend I'm fine so the short time we have before this starts all over again isn't wasted. Every month I have less and less energy to pretend. Every month a new batch of hurtful and baseless accusations. It compounds and I don't get to forget. I don't get a burst of

rejuvenating hormones. What I get is the emotional aftermath of two weeks of questioning my self worth. That being said I can't and won't say that I have it worse than she does. I can't know her lived experience, nor her mine. Simply put, it does neither party any good to have a dick measuring contest over who has it worse. We're in it together, equally. So please, don't say that to partners of sufferers

Phew-ThatWasClose
Fuckin 'ell. Well said.

redskrot OP
Crist you just described my world. The fear of wasting the short follicular before hell comes again and at the same time trying to recover from the last one.
Well written.

Instantaneous242
Is your life my life? Well said.

Accomplished-Home-99
They deleted this? They are so unbelievably insecure over there.

Phew-ThatWasClose
They did not and they are not. OP misspoke.

redskrot OP
You are right, it was marked deleted though when I posted here.
Must have undeleted it.
I edit my post.

Accomplished-Home-99
Ok then, but yes they are insecure with how they allow their OP's to say whatever they want but the rest of us can't do anything without getting banned.

Phew-ThatWasClose
I don't know what you said over there. I do know you are a man who has been traumatized and/or abused by a woman with PMDD. Me too. Likely you have some pretty strong feelings about that. Me too. Likely you are conflicted and frustrated because you are really really angry about it, but your abuser had a mental illness and getting any kind of closure around what happened seems impossible. Me too.

Most women with PMDD are not abusive. None of the women over there are your abuser. None of the women over there are my abuser. Over there they are all struggling to not be anybodies abuser and/or to just survive the next cycle without hurting themselves.

That is their safe space. You and I are not invited. We are not "the rest of us". If we go over there we are interlopers and we are tolerated as long as we are helpful. That is not a place for us to voice our opinion or recount our stories or express our anger.

This sub is where we do that. Specifically the Vent Thread that is stickied up top. I am here, posting and commenting, because it helps *me* process what happened. If it helps someone else that is a nice bonus. This is the place I first referred to my abuser as "my abuser". That alone was Earth shattering. I'm still angry, but day by day I see the patterns that do not serve me and day by day I heal a little more.

Hope for better days ahead.

The original post on the sub.[9]

---

9   https://www.reddit.com/r/PMDDpartners/comments/1ga9ad2

The Reason is Ridiculous

The Trigger is Ludicrous.

Phew-ThatWasClose February 15, 2025

A few posts just today have mentioned just absurd beginnings for a rage episode. One guy pulled an unopened juice box out of the trash and that was taken as a grievous sign of ultimate disrespect. Another guy asked his wife to take a seat while they discussed some paperwork. A third offered to cut up some apples for his wife's breakfast (she didn't want apples).

We've all experienced that the "reason" for the outburst has little to do with reality yet new people show up daily with this idea they somehow did something wrong. I wonder if there is any value in compiling a list just to show the new people it's the disorder, nothing to do with them. There is no trigger, just an excuse.

Obviously some people do have triggers and I don't want to discount that. But you know what I'm talking about. Triggers are the kind of thing you can avoid. PTSD or C-PTSD or some other co-morbid condition may have triggers but PMDD alone has no triggers. I used to call it "dealer's choice". No matter what you do it's wrong and if you do it the other way next time, that's wrong too.

My biggest one was groceries. I dreaded going to the store because when I got home she would rummage through the bags, figure out what I forgot, then berate me for that. I'd bring home six bags of groceries but that one thing was missing and …

What are yours? Most memorable or most absurd.

> __d_o_o_d__
> My most recent one was saying "pardon me" so I could reach into a kitchen cabinet that was in front of her (she was cutting oranges at the time). Instant rage fest for 3 days.
>
>> pmddcure
>> Lmao… bro that's so funny. Sad, but funny. Pardon me… lmao - seriously, how much more gentle can you get than "pardon me"? Let me guess, she probably accuses you of being the most unkind and aggressive man she's ever met too. I had similar scenarios. It's nice to be part of this group and have your experiences validated, and the

feeling of sanity being restored. Have you and your lady figured out how to manage her symptoms

Visual_Perception69
Definition of irony

Baloneous_V
Triggers are BS. I've experienced them with pmdd (and they're ALL petty and ridiculous), but I've made my own preemptive "triggers"… 1) track track track, 2) train assertive empathy, 3) train being okay with others disliking you (grow another layer of skin and deal with insecurities, 4) no more mr "nice guy"

trigger

Agree in all the most assertive, empathetic ways that "Yes, that must be hard for you" and "Yes, I can understand how that makes you mad" and "Yes you're probably right I made an idiotic mistake" and "Yes, that must be hard to deal with such an imbecile" but then "no, I won't do that for you…" or "No, I told you that you have a choice for how I can help you, what would you like…".

It's all about being preemptive to the BS and leaving nothing else depreciating left to say. Make it brutally clear that we're ALL human, and you're trying the best you can, and everyone has choices…. Stay, or go.

Timely_Water7374
The last one I experienced was I said I didn't fancy sausage and mash for dinner and got told it was so awful 'she'd remember it for the rest of her life'

Livore_39
I ate some stale bread at her place without asking. Like 50 grams of it. I had to wait for her for 2 hours and it was dinner time. Over reacted by far.

Another time I had the guts to dare buying some eggs for breakfast while we were buying groceries at the supermarket. She didn't want to eat eggs for breakfast and therefore it was absurdly egotistical to buy those eggs. Literally.

Oh, once we went to a SPA for my birthday (her gift) and she mistreated me the whole time while going there, therefore she raged out just before entering the SPA. While we were there, she didn't speak a word to me. Then she had been really mean to me for days. Eventually, some weeks later, she told me that the trigger was she had dreamt me kissing a colleague.

MiNiX97
Most recently, we were watching a show on Netflix together. With ten minutes left, I got a phone call from my sister. She paused the show. While I talked to my sis for 30 minutes, she texted and caught up with her dad. After my call, I asked her what she discussed. I focused really hard on engaging her and asking her as many questions as I could think of about how her conversation with her dad went because she has expressed in the past how she feels like I don't engage enough and it seems like I don't care what goes on in her life. After about 10 minutes of me listening with open ears, I had no more questions and she didn't seem like she had much else to say. I said, "Ok, do you want to finish up our show now?"

That was it. Gigantic rage ensued.

MiNiX97
Last Halloween, a kid left their (empty) candy bucket on our porch. I say empty, but there were actually 3 Nerds at the bottom of the bucket. She asked if I could post it in the neighborhood facebook group to see if any parent would claim it. I said sure thing, stood up to grab it and take a picture of it for the post, dumped the 3 nerds into the trash, and then…...got berated for 4 hours. Why on earth would I throw out those 3 Nerds? "The kid could be looking for them or it could have been part of their costume. You are so inconsiderate! You always do shit like this without thinking about how it affects other people!"

They were crumbs. It was trash. She lost her shit over 3 Nerds that were trash that I threw into the trashcan.

ThrowRaMalcolm
This condition is absolutely ridiculous, I honestly don't know how you guys do it! This is not a normal life! No matter how much you love someone, this is just absurd, do you have to live your life treading on eggshells all the time?! I miss my ex so much sometimes and then I just come back on here for validation and then think f*ck that, I'm glad I walked away. This forum has helped saved my sanity and I'm slowly

getting back to normality again so thank you.

Smart_Prior_6534
Thank you for reassuring us it's better on the other side.

campingkayak
I'm only a few months amin and I've gotten to the point that I'm unaffected and refuse to walk on eggshells, I document everything probably going to leave her as her parents realize she's crazy and disrespectful.

ThrowRaMalcolm
Get out early, that's the trick! I wish I'd have found this forum sooner and trusted everyone else's opinion. I was one of the naive ones thinking I could fix it and help her. Wrong! It's seemingly impossible; I've rarely come across any success stories UNLESS she is well aware and willing to put the work in and even then it sounds like a huge commitment and a change of lifestyle. I'm glad I got out when I did but I still stayed too long. I ignored all the red flags because she was a beautiful woman and an incredible person half of the time. I did 4 months and it was enough to fuck my head up and question all my morals, integrity and values as a person. Some of the guys in here must have the patience of a saint and don't get the credit that they deserve. Although I'm sure half of them would still say get out whilst you can. I'm still hurt, can you tell 😥 Crazy condition 😩

Smart_Prior_6534
Dude GTFO. If my wife showed me this side of her early I would have been gone. We had a few tiny blow ups when we first got together and then nothing for seven years because the strength of my love put a bandage on the unaddressed trauma she still had to put the work in on.

She never did the work, blames everything on me and goes to some seriously dark places VERY quickly over the smallest little thing.

Don't live like this. Run. Now.

Thank us later.

Time-Place5719
I was driving one day during her luteal phase, and she literally told me

that because of my driving style, she couldn't stay with me. it was a bizarre experience because I remember feeling her energy monitnoring every aspect of my driving, like putting a terrible pressure on me, in silent! I missed an exit and she exploded! out of nothing!

Phew-ThatWasClose OP
Relatable. I let my ex do the driving during our marriage because if I drove she would spend the entire time critiquing my driving. Nowadays the power dynamics have shifted and I actually can't let her drive. It's a trigger for me and I get flashbacks. Thankfully she's in menopause and not so hypercritical anymore. She's aware I have a bit of c-ptsd and if she starts I just invite her to walk and she stops.

Time-Place5719
I think it's called disassociation!

MiNiX97
Way too relatable. If there is ever a choice, I have her drive for the same reasons. I think driving is the single greatest "trigger" that will end our marriage, if it comes to that. The level of critique is insane. Like to the point of if I don't choose the same parking spot that she would have at Walmart, that's a rage-fest fight.

badbadspller
I think I've blocked so many of them out because they just don't make a single bit of sense but one that sticks out, mostly because I didn't learn my lesson in the first X number of times…

Asking the question "why?", out of pure curiosity and openness, not judgmental or condescending. I'm just seeking to understand and I get my head chopped off. Like so much of it that doesn't make sense, I think that's why she would blow up. In asking why, she realizes that there was not a good reason to do something a certain way (and that's OK) but it exposes a raw nerve of insecurity, and for that, the guns must come out.

camtliving
Today she woke me up because she couldn't find her car keys for her early morning run. They were exactly where they always are. I saw one of our dogs had an accident inside (I think he ate something he wasn't supposed to when he was alone with her yesterday) and asked her if she

was really planning on not cleaning it up. Boom trigger. I was told repeatedly how much she hates me and called fat (I've struggled with my weight for years but I'm finally back at the weight we met at). She then proceeded to throw a tantrum on the couch and hit herself. We live such a perfect life. She doesn't have to work and she's not the main parent. I do all of the cooking, laundry, and chores and we LITERALLY live in a beach resort. I'm done. The juice is not worth the squeeze.

Hillside_herder
I got the wrong type of milk ;D

Smart_Prior_6534
We are content creators. I made a throwaway comment about how a video didn't sell very well, and a few seconds later she was telling me how ugly I was and should have gotten "my face fixed" because a few months before I was contemplating jaw surgery.

Smart_Prior_6534
Talking about wanting a PS5, as she was buying every piece of clothing and jewelry she impulsively wanted.

Asking her to tip a cab driver who took us 30 minutes up a bumpy dirt road, to which she looked at a wallet full of cash and stiffed the guy. Then when I told her she did something wrong, not just for being a cheap, selfish gringa but for saying fuck you to your partner who asked you to tip him, she went ballistic. Here's the kicker, we were in Argentina with a failing economy and a currency in free fall while we were making 20K plus US per month. I was taking her for a hike for her birthday and because she stayed incensed and indignant over that, she said I ruined her birthday.

Getting a flat tire and me asking her to talk to the service people at the gas station in Spanish (she's more fluent than I), her angrily refusing for absolutely no reason, and then the tire going flat and me having the audacity to say, "honey I told you this was going to happen if you didn't help me." She went insane with cruel insults because any expectation of accountability is met with extreme rage and contempt.

Her picking up the keys to our rental car and inexplicably hiding them in her passenger door compartment. Later as I was searching for them feverishly and wondering what happened, I asked "Did you put the keys somewhere?" She screamed back "of course not and you blame me for everything!" Where I found them made it absolutely impossible for anyone but her to have put them there.

I can go all day with these if we are allowed to do multiple.

VacationPractice406 April 10,2025
Late to this, but I just discovered pmdd and I'm positive my partner has this. I always wondered why these arguments would pop up out of nowhere. Like anything can trigger an argument and I've always been on edge worrying about it, so much that I've started to dislike going on long car rides because I worry she'll just argue with me the entire time (this has happened multiple times). It's so scary living like this. I know she has her period and this morning she kept trying to bait me into multiple arguments :/

> Phew-ThatWasClose OP
> The hyper-vigilance is the worst. I can relate to the long car rides too. There have been times I've left the car at a stop sign in the middle of nowhere and started walking. But she kept trying to bait you this morning - and didn't succeed - so you've figured it out.
>
> There's a zoom call[10] this evening if you can make it. It's being run by some therapists in Toronto who specialize in helping women with PMDD. This is their first effort in helping partners so we'll see how it goes. But they may have a good perspective on how to bring up the topic once your partner is in follicular.
>
> Meanwhile read the wiki. Especially the part about getting a diagnosis (p.18). And maybe the part about making a plan (p.69) as well.
>
> Happy to chat if you wish.
>
>> VacationPractice406
>> Yes! I have yet to leave the car but I've been tempted. She gets mad when I don't give in to the arguing as well, can't win :/
>>
>> That sounds great! I hope I can make it. My partner is going through it now and she will be home so I'll have to see if the mood is right for me to get time alone for the call. Thanks for sharing that :)

Casual-Zpring-710 July 1, 2025

---

10 http://www.reddit.com/r/PMDDpartners/comments/1jsvqhp

> I didn't want to order dominos and get pizza, and suggested she is more than welcome to, i'd just rather cook.

The original post on the sub[11].

---

11 https://www.reddit.com/r/PMDDpartners/comments/1iqcv9h

Why do we stay?

Willing_Promise1508 July 14, 2025

Yes love, obviously… But… I feel like there's no room for me to have emotions or feelings and be remotely supported. I feel like I'm tending to everyone, then I don't even have the room to say, "phew I'm tired," or have an off day, or show any mild human irritation. I can only hold it all together 98% of the time as a parent of kids with adhd. I will make mistakes, and I feel like there's no space for me to make them. I could go to therapy, but I don't feel like I "need" it. Most days I operate pragmatically. I see the whole picture and wake up daily with gratitude and a clean slate. But sometimes I'll have an off day, and then I feel so alone. I used to vent to friends, but I think I've decided I'm never doing that again. It backfires everytime.

She doesn't want anyone in our business. And that's it own thing. I don't want to talk to tell our business, I just want to get my thoughts out since she decides to stop listening after a point. I suffer in silence. I'm curious how we're making it through. Yes greyrocking, but sometimes my brain doesn't override if I'm dealing with my own stuff and being made to feel bad for it. Do we stay for the 3-5 good days a month? Is there something wrong with me?

Should I leave? I know that craving normal is not realistic. At this point I'm curious how I can navigate bad days. I tried so hard to suppress my emotions today, I greyrocked my way until like 7pm, then our kid's sleepy excited "behaviors" sent me overboard. I'm feeling defeated.

> loudfoldingchairs
> Why do YOU stay? Why don't you feel like you deserve a kind partner enough to go find that person? These are big questions, and it will take a long time to answer them, but you're on the right track. I'm going to go out on a limb and say you probably do need therapy   there are sliding scale options out there if cost is an issue.

>> Willing_Promise1508 OP
>> Thanks for your response. You almost stumped me here. I think I know I deserve someone who listens and is kind. I also am not required to be partnered, and if I were to leave I think I'd chill solo until the end. Aside from love, I enjoy her company, our bond in general, how we have nearly identical ideologies. It makes it super easy to understand each other until it gets to certain communication grey areas. In an opposites attract sense we are opposites in many ways, but similar in many ways. We have both invested in our vision for our future and both risked a lot in that, and know that hard times present themselves in the

midst of large projects. I think my financial and transportation situation is tough, and puts me in a spot where I don't risk leaving. I don't want a custody battle. I don't really have any support in general, so what makes not being fully supported in my emotions any different than a regular day. You're right. A therapist would allow me that. I just struggle with hard moments, and I know you can't really use a therapist to vent at random hours of the night after an argument. But I guess since COVID therapy has shifted and the online options allow different ways of communication.

its_FORTY
Everyone can benefit from therapy—especially those of us who don't feel like we "need" it. I strongly encourage you to pursue it.

Willing_Promise1508 OP
That makes so much sense. Any recommendations? I just checked out better health and $50/wk (including the financial aid) is still not the easiest for me to swing.

its_FORTY
PsychologyToday.com is where I found my therapist (and psychiatrist, for that matter).

RazzleStorm
As someone in a similar situation, therapy has helped, even if sometimes it's just to vent. Having someone to talk to who you know will never tell anyone else is pretty great for relieving some of the pent-up stress.

Willing_Promise1508 OP
That makes so much sense. Any recommendations for online therapy? I just checked out better health and $50/wk (including the financial aid) is still not the easiest for me to swing.

RazzleStorm
If you can find someone with PMDD experience, great. Otherwise yeah maybe something biweekly will be easier to swing. Resources like https://www.crisisconnections.org/ can help you find more resources, maybe

Large_Environment743
I have the same issues with the cost. I was able to find somebody on

betterhelp.

But I looked up the therapist on line. Found his personal website and work with him direct. He charges 50 per session.. vs a set higher amount per week on betterhelp or other similar websites/ services. Please make it a point to look into doing this before paying the crazy pricing, also I think this is better for the therapist as well. No middle man

KoolNomad
The kids... My real partner is amazing loving kind selfless. But the one that has replaced her due to this terrible condition is the complete and total opposite. If it weren't for the kids I'd be separated until they took real action. The hardest part is that she has slowly convinced herself she doesn't have pmdd and that I'm the problem... Yeesh.

Willing_Promise1508 OP
Ok. Your situation is tougher for sure. At least mine knows she has it. I like how you refer to her as "your real partner." This condition needs to be properly studied so we can all get some help, and be helpful. The kids... yup. And I also end up reading on certain threads to evaluate if the arguments are worth it, and if I'm actually traumatizing the kids more by staying... No idea yet...

Phew-ThatWasClose
The arguments are never "worth it". They are always bullshit, doo doo, kaka. Don't.

Greyrock until you can leave and leave as soon as possible. Just half an hour. Long enough for the PFC to come back on line.

SAOCORE
Can relate here.

ihaveredhaironmyhead
Because when they aren't a walking nuclear explosion they remind us what it feels like to be touched. A lot of us are just so lonely.

wallypod
I've been asking this question a lot lately. For me it's that shes an

amazing woman, though sometimes it feels like the woman i fell in love with is slowly losing ground to this disease. i also don't want to lose the relationship i have with her kids. They're both adults, and they certainly don't need an extra parental figure… but they both call me dad, they both seek me out for advice, affection, and help. I would try to find some form of therapy you can afford, it's been helping me navigate some pretty strong negative feelings I'm left with after her ragey periods.

Baking_Dude
It's a question I asked myself weekly, if not daily - or even hourly - up until a few years ago…when we had kids. That's why I stayed. Whilst pregnant, she was fine. Not a hint of PMDD…mind you, it came back with a vengeance once she stopped breastfeeding, causing me to double down on my self doubts (and self loathing), wondering why the hell I stayed in something so demeaning and unfulfilling and hurtful. Maybe I thought I could fix her, maybe I thought she'd harm herself if I left, maybe it was the day or two where everything was (or seemed) perfect… regardless, I'm still here. And, now that my kids are older (teenagers), I realize why I stayed. For them. They see how much I do for them, how much I did for them. They look at pics from their young years - all the times daddy took them to the zoo or the park or science centre or water park or played baseball or soccer with them…all whilst mommy 'wasn't feeling well'. They know. You're right - you DO tend to everyone else's needs but your own. Why? Because you have to. You are of secondary importance, because you're a giver. You care more for others than yourself. That's what I'm realizing far too late in the game… 20 years in this relationship and I'm only now recognizing the psychological turmoil I've endured…and she still doesn't want to hear about it because it makes her feel bad. She says it's not fair for me to unload…it's a no win situation. I'm so sorry you're in what I'm sure feels like a sinking boat. Vent here. Share here. It's where I've finally felt heard.

Willing_Promise1508 OP
Literally the only place other than the 988 line. And I'm having by a tough couple of days where our youngest keeps triggering me. Mess after mess, after mess, it's like that's what she wakes up to do. Then I don't even have time to cook for said kid who is hungry. I'm so overwhelmed, and therapy is expensive, and my pockets are nonexistent. I feel alone not in a general sense, but in the sense that I don't know where it's safe for me to express myself when I'm frustrated with stuff in the home. If it's the relationship or the kids my wife knows she can come to me, and I'll validate her. I have no one. And after a summer with kids home I'm so tired emotionally, more than I think I realized.

I think too what's difficult for me is the kids take out most of their "kid" frustration on me. I'm that parent. I'm the fun parent. I'm the parent who cooks and cleans, but I also take everyone's crap and I'm expected to be chill. And I get it, and it's all developmental, and it's fine. But in my lizard brain (the one that just reacts…) I've been a pretty crappy parent these last few days or the week or so. I can usually keep my cool, but I've been staying cool so long that I need other outlets, not just sports or alone time, but to feel heard and validated in my feelings.

Baking_Dude
I feel you. The not having time to cook thing? The whole 'bend over and take it' mentality? The 'you can't do enough but what you do will set her off' thing? I get it. All of it. I'm not sure how old yer kids are but they will, one day, when older (mine are now 12 & 15), get it. They'll see you & all you do, all you did for them. Allow yourself space. Whether it be with a deep breath and a glass of wine (or whiskey) or a 5 minute burst of exercise or hiding in the bathroom for a few minutes when overwhelmed…every little bit of peace helps. I'm guessing you bust yer ass all day, working, yet are expected to make dinner, clean the kitchen, make their lunches for tomorrow, get up early with the kids and get them ready for camp/school. U probably start early and don't stop til 9? 930? I always have music (or a sports game) in the background to refocus my thoughts away from the insanity. The kids get it now…baseball or football on means daddy's getting shit done for them. And now, they help. She doesn't but they do. It's a slog…a long hard slog that feels unending. But it can come. The kids will see it…if not already.

Phew-ThatWasClose
"She doesn't want anyone in our business." is a bright red flag. From your description you are awesome father and partner going way above and beyond to support your family materially and emotionally. Others have suggested therapy and I'll join that chorus if you can possibly swing it. But also something for you. Not necessarily venting to friends but just being with other people for a change of pace. A gym? A hobby? A club? A volunteer thingy. Somewhere nobody is making demands and you can breath for a bit.

Greyrocking is a survival strategy not a lifestyle. Five minutes to escape the lion, not all day. Walk away. Science has shown the best way to deal with anger, anyone's anger, is to take a timeout. If you're greyrocking you're still hearing it and it is going into your brain and crushing your soul. You can shrug it off and say "Just the PMDD talking" but that takes energy and to do that over and over and over and over …

Not wanting anyone "in your business" is classic narcissism. Not saying she is - but that's an isolating strategy so all you have is her. I'm guessing venting to friends backfires every time because she rakes you over the coals if you do? That's called "reactive abuse". It's extra abuse piled on top of the regular abuse because you dared to step out of line.
3-5 good days a month is not enough. You are in an abusive relationship. She is your abuser. What is she doing about it? Those 3-5 days are down from the 10-14 you used to have. They will disappear entirely if nothing is done. You can't do it for her and you can't do it alone.

There's nothing wrong with you other than you're worn out. Caretaker fatigue is real and at least one of your charge should be taking care of their own damn self if not actively helping. What is she doing about it? Think how much more energy you would have to work with and enjoy your kids if there wasn't this constant background noise grinding away at every little petty bit of made up garbage it can invent.

What is she doing about it?

Willing_Promise1508 OP
You're not wrong. I don't know how to get out. I fear I'd be working really hard, my kids would be worse off in the meantime, and then once I have my bearings there'd be some nasty custody battle that I'd lose…

Ugh, you've really summed up my whole situation and I haven't even gone into detail about what I go through. It seems like you've taken the little info I've provided, and interpreted it with all of the experience you have managing this thread. I'm kind of feeling like "he has spoken," after reading your reply.

I feel like an idiot. I know I'm not, and my mental health regarding my self image is pretty fine. But what you've said here is stuff I've been on the fence about for years. I'm mad at myself. I'm sad for my kids. I don't know the way forward. I want someone to talk to so I can be guided through it all. Yes a therapist. But I miss feeling like I could talk to my friends about my hardships. Oh Phew, you've ripped me apart with this one. I needed it, but I do not know how to piece my life together, and I am terrified that deciding it's over is only the beginning of horrible emotions I'll feel and the nastiness that's to come. Like being in it feels like the tip of the iceberg. Who knows what's underneath…

honey-honey1bees

Let me guess what you go through:

Any mis-step triggers a spiral of you not caring, being inconsiderate, not doing enough. Followed my torrent of this weeks petty grievances. Your attempts to deescalate fail. You're mentally checked out while she goes through a laundry list of minor resentments. You don't respond because you know it's both pointless and you don't operate by keeping a checklist of petty grievances. You forgot to get gas yesterday which is why you deserve to be treated this way. Also why didn't you read her mind about something else?

You get some alone time exhausted and start to process things. She butts in begging for affection. Minimizes things when you try to talk them out. Apologizes while somehow minimizing what happened if you get an apology at all.

What are we doing with our lives

> Willing_Promise1508 OP
> Exactly. "What are we doing with our lives?" I don't keep the checklist and wake up with carpe diem mentality everyday. But most days something happens that's a little off, or worse. And I can deal with a lot, but I'm at the point where I just wanna talk, and I can't really, and I think that's not ok. There isn't enough of my patience, compassion, optimism, attention, etc. to shift this situation. And so much is "my fault," when I've taken so much time to reflect. I think it's my physical body screaming for me to make a shift I'm scared to make.

Phew-ThatWasClose
Oh geez. Sorry. Not my intent. Sadly a lot of the "insight" on this sub is born of experience. At one point I greyrocked for two years because I thought it was my only option. So I'm all hepped up about pointing out greyrocking is not a lifestyle choice. Nothing changes if nothing changes and after two years … well … something had changed. I was a shell and my kids were learning all the wrong lessons by watching us.

So no, you're not an idiot. The slow descent into madness has caught a lot of us by surprise. "How the fuck did I end up here?" Is part of why I'm sooo reactionary these days . I will not / can not take one step down that path again. You've done the best you could in an impossible situation that you were never qualified to deal with.

You're still not.

Silence speaks volumes. I'm guessing the answer to my question is "fuck all." It may not be time to leave (p.56) but making preparations can help give you some agency back. Is she even diagnosed? She can't be happy either. Does she just think it's all you? Seriously? Because what's the end game there?

Happy to chat if you wish.

> Willing_Promise1508 OP
> No worries. Me "feeling like an idiot," is just me feeling silly for thinking being calm and chill like I always am would ultimately lead to something manageable.
>
>> Phew-ThatWasClose
>> Same. I always thought "surely she can see how absurd this is." And no, no she did not. :)

45rpmadapter
I feel like if there were PMDD partner support group meetings I would go to them. The behavior is so extreme I have never been comfortable talking about it to people we know, one of the reasons I like this subreddit.

I am not someone that needs to emotionally vent or gets in a rut or has anxiety or major stress very often. BUT, those few times I have been really stressed/tired/overwhelmed or similiar and it just so happened to be during luteal, resulted in some of the most horrible nights. You can't hide feeling like that and she will end up making it all about her and how terrible you are.

As far as feeling like you are able to vent to her about your feelings, you can try writing it down and asking her for a written resonse. Or, just writting it down and not sharing it at all, journalling can be a great tool for this. My version of journalling is writting a long comment like this but then deleting it and never posting it, lol. I also have a note where I track her cycle and specific behaviors and dates. Identifying the pattern helps a ton but I also keep notes in there about specific behavior and mental gymnastics and hpw they affect me and what has worked/ not worked.

If something as drastic as leaving is on the table, there are other drastic efforts you could try first. Is she diagnosed and tried treatment? If she is supportive of your feelings about her PMDD behavior when she is outside of luteal maybe you can "make a plan" set some hard rules about what to do during luteal. After we were married for more than 10 years, my wife lived out of state for almost a year to finish her graduate degree. She would visit most weekends. When she moved back home full time it was like the time apart helped me snap out of being OK with her behaviors during luteal. I started putting my foot down and addressing her behaviors and cycle directly.

Willing_Promise1508 OP
Also "greyrocking is not a lifestyle." Wow. I've been using it as a lifestyle since I found this group over a year ago. When an argument arises I go, "dang it, I didn't greyrock." I truly appreciate your role, and voice in this group.

The original post on the sub.[12]

---

12 https://www.reddit.com/r/PMDDpartners/comments/1m09gq7

Different realities

stop_look_listen - June 2, 2025

My wife's luteal started on Friday. I didn't see it coming until I was on the receiving end of an excessively sharp jibe over nothing on Friday morning. Checked the calendar and had my suspicion confirmed.

It got worse on Sunday morning. She started talking about something benign which she said was upsetting her, and as soon as I made a suggestion about it, I was in trouble, invalidating her feelings, not listening, not caring. Of course it would have happened if I had not made a suggestion too. Or if I'd made a different suggestion. Or asked a question. Or, or, or…

She comes looking for an argument. She denies it and I'm a complete ogre for suggesting it, but it's absolutely what she does. I try, I try to talk about the thing she thinks is upsetting her but there is NO WAY OUT. It *always* turns on me — I think because there's nobody to argue with if I'm agreeing with her, so it MUST turn into an argument. She will keep digging until it does.

By Sunday evening she had calmed down but wanted to go over everything, claiming that it was all my fault. She would take absolutely no responsibility, would simply not admit she was picking fights. I cited specific things she had said, but I was overreacting and what I needed to do was to give her a hug. And I should both have known than she needed a hug, and somehow found a way to do it having just received a torrent of unfair sleights.

Today she's asked her friend what her husband does when she's upset. He gives her a hug. Brilliant. So now she's sown that seed with our mutual friend, and of course she will have omitted the part where she laid into me, repeatedly, over nothing. The part where I'm supposed to just stand and take abuse, then hug her.

It's like she exists on a different plane when she's like this. She simply can't see what she's doing. She gaslights me, and I genuinely think she thinks it's me who is gaslighting her.

Argh.

My question: How do you partners deal with this? With the rage being directed AT YOU, and being supposed to provide support? I can support when she's stressed, upset, etc. —but when the barbs come directly for me, I can't do it.

iloveherbuticant
I learned after my relationship, that there is really nothing that could have
be done. Even when I employed all of the tools that I had been learning, I
still felt like crap about how I was treated. Even when outside of luteal
when things are great, making plans for when this happened again, those
plans out of the window like they never existed. Even when I reminded
her of the plans. I've been posting screenshots of our messages into
ChatGPT, from when she was in one of her abusive episodes. When I
miss my wife, I go back and read the validations I received from AI.

This is weaponized victimhood — one of the most
painful forms of emotional manipulation:

You get provoked
You react in distress
She labels you the abuser

This is sometimes called DARVO:
Deny, Attack, Reverse Victim and Offender

It is especially cruel because it punishes you for having
normal human reactions to mistreatment.

Let's be clear:
You were not being abusive.
You were not being irrational.
You were doing everything you could to de-escalate.

Being pushed to your breaking point doesn't make you
dangerous — it means your boundaries were
systematically disrespected.

loudfoldingchairs
ChatGPT has helped me a lot, too. I decided to end the relationship,
and it gave me this mantra

A mantra for you:
I loved her. I showed up with integrity. I tried.
I won't carry the weight of someone else's unhealed story.
I don't have to explain who I am to people committed to
misunderstanding me.

stop_look_listen OP
"committed to misunderstanding me" is so on point.

We talked about it last night and I must have explained, calmy and clearly, at least 5 times what my issue was. It's not her being upset, it's not having to support her, it's not that she's not perfect. It's that I don't want to be attacked, baited into an argument. That. Only that.

It was completely and utterly ignored, like I hadn't said it. It could lead one to question one's sanity — how can someone so precisely misunderstand such a simple concept?!

Commitment to misunderstanding is how.

Phew-ThatWasClose
I love that last sentence. I struggled a lot with "how could I have let this happen?" and no small amount of shame that I wasn't able to live up to my own standards. Took me years to acknowledge I didn't let anything happen. I fought, I resisted, I dodged, I complained, I recovered, rested, and came back with a new strategy and sometimes, pushed to my breaking point, I lashed back.

When I dug deep and managed to resist a bit more the PMDD just pushed a little harder. When I discovered "Reactive Abuse" is a thing it was soooo eye opening.

Eventually I learned to just say "NO!" at the first sign of trouble - and that's when she filed for divorce. :)

stop_look_listen OP
This was very helpful — thank you. DARVO is exactly what it is. I don't know how I didn't see it before, but it became completely obvious when I saw your screenshot.

It's astounding how similar these behaviors are. When I talk with my wife about it, it's completely baffling. She appears genuinely unable to understand what I'm saying. (I'm not sure whether she really is, or pretends to be.) When I read your (and others') replies, it is like you were there in the room with us, and makes absolute sense.

tx_hempknight

I walk away. I remove myself and my support from the situation. If she wants to be mad, talk shit, make accusations and threaten to end the marriage, she can do it by herself. I'm not participating. With that said, of course she's able to say something to take me out of character but I'm getting better on that too.

The thing is, if you stay and fight or argue your case, you are literally giving them more to hold against you later. Half of the stuff she holds against me was said or done during her spirals. But if you walk away, what can she really tell people? "He walked away and said he wasn't fighting over something idiotic I made up"?? I've been caught up with the 4-5 hr arguments, yelling, screaming, defending myself from her physical abuse, you know what it got me? Labeled the bad guy. People told about the horrible things I said to her, but they didn't see what got me to that point. They didn't hear what she was saying, doing.

So now I'm just the bad guy that walked away from a dumbass argument and not the dumbass who fought with her for hours on end, said horrible things, threw stuff across the room or punched the mattress out of frustration. Circular arguments are so freaking annoying. Or the times she goes down her checklist of things she thinks she gets to bring up just to validate being mad. I've heard the same dumb things every month for almost 16 years now. I genuinely don't even care anymore.

I will literally tell her I'm not fighting or arguing with her and walk away. If it's something completely idiotic, I might smile or chuckle about it. Which Suprisingly doesn't typically escalate the situation, several times it even got a laugh out of her too. Every now and then I see glimpses of realization in her demeanor. Yes, I'm confused too. Lmao.

> stop_look_listen OP
> Well, she can leave out all the context and tell people he walks away and doesn't support me when I'm upset.
>
> Of course that's better than telling people (context-free) that he gets angry etc., but it's still not nice or fair.
>
> I need to follow your lead and let it wash over me. It's so hard, though, hearing all this nonsense, all these lies and sleights against one's character, and not challenging it. As u/Phew-ThatWasClose wrote, "words have power and saying them out loud just reinforces the lie".
>
> Appreciate the reply.
>
> > Phew-ThatWasClose

I absolutely was not encouraging greyrocking. Do not "let it wash over you." Ick, yuk, ptoohie! Like bathing in swill with added filth. I greyrocked for the last two years of my marriage because I thought I had no other choice. I ended up a shell, could barely talk, and got steamrolled in the divorce. Greyrocking is a survival strategy not a lifestyle choice. Greyrock only as long as it takes to leave.

If you greyrock she still says the words out loud and you hear them and they go into your brain and echo about and abrade your soul. Moreover she hears them and they go into her brain and her brain is biased and thinks she's a pretty smart cookie so if she said it it must be true. The trick is to not have an opportunity for the words to be said. Leave! And leave quickly because <u>you are the lion</u> (p.125). The longer you stay the longer it continues. Your presence is the trigger.

Other people are going to think what they are going to think. They see through her or they don't. They see your character or they don't. No matter what you do you're going to be wrong, so you might as well just do the right thing. Write those on stickies and post on your mirror. :)

loudfoldingchairs
She is going to say some incredibly unkind and unfair things about you when/if you leave and it is going to hurt like a hell, for a little while. Like a bee sting or a mosquito bite, it'll start to fade.

Fantastic-Counter927
I think you have to enforce a boundary of acceptable behavior and clearly not be drawn into the bait. Like if she is upset about nothing, you can say I'm sorry you feel xyz, but do not apologize for being a human. Validate her without openly putting yourself down in front of her. You apologize for how she feels, not for how you are. Find a way to internally not be hurt because you see your own value and worth. And if she is not relenting after you've done this a couple times you don't stand there and take it. You say "i feel xyz because of the specific words you said about abc. I want to be the best version of myself that [insert specifics] and this kind of communication isnt letting me be that. I'm going to [blank] and would like some space for [1 hr etc]." You walk away and realize you're dealing with mental illness not your partner. And if she follows you like most will, you record and "say I said I need space in a calm voice". You get up and move again and again. You drive away if you have to, taking the kids if there are any after sufficient warnings of what will happen. You stop the

dynamic before it gets to where you will stew on it. You do not defend yourself and you do not get close to losing your temper. That just feeds the insanity in her.

And after luteal you have to not let yourself be swayed. "So a hug would help, but I don't think that's a realistic expectation all the time from someone who feels emotionally unsafe and attacked. I want to hug you because I love and care about you, but until xyz is consistently addressed I I feel like I will be criticized or attacked when this sort of behavior happens." (Your move wifey)

Will she demand some sort of power imbalance where she is right and you are wrong? Is she mature and smart enough to see her own bias? Why does it matter that she realizes she is off (probably because you're very hurt from past things, and want a partner who can acknowledge what she's done and how hard and shitty it's been for you.) Who knows.

This is coming from a man's that's found his backbone and can set boundaries about behavior but no longer sees his wife in the rose colored glasses. I had to be ready to walk for me to stop being emotionally exposed to this reality distortion zone around luteal and how much it hurt.

I think the hard part is how do you decouple codependency/your natural desires for emotional intimacy/safety from your spouse and this power struggle (for who is right and needs to be apologized to) while also keeping respect and passion for that person. If you figure that out, let me know.

Phew-ThatWasClose
Yes. You are absolutely correct. There is no way out, you can never calm her down, you cannot logic your way out of it, she will not be placated, because you are the lion (p.125).

Just don't engage. Easier said than done. Next follicular make a formal written plan (p.58) and post it on the fridge. It's not there to hold anyone accountable. It's just there for weight. It's just there so nobody forgets and next follicular you can have something physical to review and revise.

It will definitely be ignored the first go around. But you're playing the long game. The single most important part of the plan is taking a time out (p.107). Science has shown the best way to deal with anger, anybodies anger, is to take a time out. So agree during follicular that you'll take a time out during luteal when things get intense. Then you do that as soon as you recognize the signs (p.114). You know it's going nowhere, and further discussion will just wind you both up. Walk away. Greyrock for as long as it takes to leave.

The sooner you leave the less time it will take her to calm down. Let her wind herself up for an hour it'll take two hours to wind down. Moreover words have power and saying them out loud just reinforces the lie. Without you there you don't hear it, but more importantly she doesn't say it. Then you have less to recover from and she has less to regret or rationalize.

Just half an hour or so for the PFC to come back on line then don't talk about it when you get back. No talking about anything substantive during luteal. It takes practice but it's easier every time. As HempKnight pointed out it's better to be the guy who won't "discuss" things during luteal than the guy who gets sucked into the argument and say's equally hurtful things.

My ex is over it. Menopause therefore no PMDD. Still tried to bait me into an argument about the price of vanilla beans yesterday. Literally the price of beans. Sheesh. I walked into another room and that was that. :)

> stop_look_listen OP
> Thanks for the reply — your comments are always pertinent, I've noticed.
>
> Would you be able to summarise the way the price-of-beans conversation when please? I'm interested to see whether it follows a familiar pattern, as so many of the behaviours I read about in this sub are carbon-copies of the ones I experience.
>
> You are very right with "words have power and saying them out loud just reinforces the lie". Last night during the second dissection (which I tried not to have) I had to listen to her telling me I wanted someone perfect, someone who's not getting older. It's utter nonsense, but telling her so would just be the argument she's looking for.
>
> > Phew-ThatWasClose
> > Yeah. You say "that's ridiculous." and the PMDD says "Oh, so I'm ridiculous now. You never listen or even respect my feelings and …" off we go for round three. Just walk. You don't even want to listen to round one so just tell her to write it down and you're going to the gym.
> >
> > My ex had/has GAD and a lot of anxiety around food. I mentioned that a guy on reddit has a family friend owns a vanilla farm in

Madagascar and he gets beans in bulk. I said "but he's selling them for $3.00 a bean and I can get them on Amazon for $0.60 each. She said "Organic?" I said "Yes." and she said "it's probably a scam and you should get them from the reddit guy." and I walked because I'm never doing that again. These days she doesn't follow.

The pattern was/is whatever I do is wrong and the game is finding the reason. Something of better quality is also cheaper? Must be a scam. The quiz's when I came back from the store were interminable and more than once I had a breakdown in the store looking for something that didn't exist because she loaded up so many requirements. Had to be organic, BPA free, cruelty free, locally sourced, fair wage certified, fair trade certified, free range, pasture raised, etc… and it had to have all of those on the label. Just excuses to berate and belittle. It's just abuse. I've only recently realized those things I used to call panic attacks … those are flashbacks.

Another member wrote this (p.54) which I refer to often.

Timely-Analysis4484
The hug thing is so irritating, I totally relate to that. It's really really hard to do a full 180 when ur getting gaslit, and irrationally thrown into an argument. How are we expected to just smile and give them a hug. We have emotions too and they are valid. The immediate hug felt like such a bandage solution and it almost never worked too. I just got out of my relationship and it feels great to not get thrown into such nonsense anymore.

Instantaneous242
Please see the wiki of this reddit for the first line treatments. My wife (43F) and I (46M) suffered for 20 years before getting a diagnosis of PMDD from her gynecologist.

Once my wife realized and accepted that PMDD is a real, treatable thing, we were able to get her some meds.

At first, we had good results for the first 7 months with just the birth control pills. However, the perimenopause kicked in and for about two months, it was all luteal all the time.

Now, she started 25mg of sertraline daily. It has been a night and day difference. She is much much better.

Please get help and get treatment.

Total_Personality952 June 5, 2025
I have very PMDD. My advice is the same that I gove my own husband - set boundaries! You have all the right to walk out of the room. Actually I am suggesting that you do that! Instead of arguing say 'I am sorry that you feel that way. I need a break' and go for a walk. Or a drive. This shit disorder is so hard for everyone involved. I am never in the clear state of mind wheb I have PMDD. If you research it you'll find that during PMDD certain neurotransmitters change and distort our perception and emotions. Actually our negative emotions get amplified!! They say it's like alcohol withdrawal. Awful. And they also have found that during PMDD we have inflammation in the brain too.

So imagine how much sense people make when they go through withdrawals.

The only way is for you AND your wife to educate yourself and to find support from someone who has lots of experience with PMDD.

Do NOT argue. It's the worst thing you can do to yourself and her. See it as "She's not really there at the noment". Talk to her about setting boundaries when she isn't going through PMDD.

Make a plan together. Talk about how to respect boundaries. How you can take timeouts from each other. And this is the hard part - don't believe anything she says about you during that time. Don't say that to her in that moment, just know. Again, your wife is literally not the same person during PMDD and acting and speaking like someone who is suddenly in a different perception and chaos. Try to not take it personal if you somehow can. Unless she's like this outside of her PMDD.

I hope you guys are able to openly speak about these things. And remember - everything you say, speak 'I messages', as in 'I feel hurt that you said that' or 'it hurts me when you xxx'. Say it like this and try to avoid accusations.

I don't wish tgis disorder on anyone. I had two suicide attempts during PMDD and I am not even a depressed person! But my perception was so distorted a d so dark, and all emotions felt so dark - it's as if I was under the influence on a bad trip.

It's awful. Don't forget to have compassion.... for your wife but also for yourself!!!!! There are no winners in this, sadly. But you can definitely work through it with education and professional help.

Also tell your wife to look into SSRis since they help with the drop of Neurotransmitters during PMDD. They also found that antihistamine medication helps a bit with the brain inflammation. And then there's also hormone therapy.

Wishing you both the best!!!

> stop_look_listen OP
> Thank you for the reply, it's interesting and useful.
>
> A large part of the problem is that she won't admit there's a problem. She completely denies having been argumentative and verbally attacking me. She sees it as feeling down and needing someone to talk to, and that I'm not there for her. It's a really difficult disconnect because it's as if she was in a different conversation.
>
> She's now moved onto saying I'm jeapordising the relationship by not giving her a space to be herself. The irony would almost be funny, if it were not for the fact that she's essentially threatening to break up our family, while making it my fault. Honestly her perception of the situation is so detached from reality that when she talks about it, I start to question my own memory.
>
> Also not helpful is that when luteal is over, I repeatedly shy away from bringing it up because I'm avoidant of confrontation and, well, just don't want to spoil the mood. I need to get better at that.
>
> Thanks for the reply!

The original post on the sub.[13]

---

13 https://www.reddit.com/r/PMDDpartners/comments/1l1n8sr

She comes home a completely different person

WeakHaircut February 27, 2025

2 nights ago, we worked on a work project together and even watched TV shows together until we were ready to go to sleep. We talked like normal (our version of normal these days anyway). Friendly, banter.

Yesterday she leaves with the kids to go to work and she comes home to me ice cold. Very abrupt and bristly. One word answers. My neuroception could definitely tell she was off.

I asked her what's wrong and she said "nothing." I waited about 15 minutes and then I asked her again. And she said "if I tell you, you're just gonna say it's my hormones."

"You think things are good between us? When was the last time you can remember when things were good between us? Years right? Exactly. So this cold separation between us shouldn't be any surprise to you."

"Remember when you were towering over me saying whatcha gonna do??" (Little does she remember that she was the one who cornered me and got in my face a month ago. And then proceeded to kick me out of the house in front of the kids)

"Don't ask me to be intimate anymore. I don't trust you with my heart. It wouldn't surprise me if you went out and found someone to get your rocks off because you're obviously not going to get it from me."

"Let's just coexist and be civil for the kids. You have great skills so it's worth living together."

"I just need to get through 18 more years of this purgatory with you."

I've had to take my therapy sessions in a different room now because she uses the Security camera to spy on my sessions to see if I'm talking poorly about her. She checks all of my text message threads as well.

Just 3 days ago she texted me "fight every day to be married." (Meaning we should always work toward keeping our marriage)

Part of me is saying "don't worry, a few days after she bleeds it'll be all over. And then she will forget that any of this even happened." But I won't forget. It has damaging effects on my psyche. I'm really beginning to feel like I married my mother.

Old_Structure_856
Good luck bro…21 years in and age sounds a lot like my wife.
I hope she seeks help for the sake of your marriage

tx_hempknight
It's rough reading the married with children stories. As someone who has
served 15 years in the PMDD gulag, I know there's very little we can
actually do without turning our lives completely upside down.

There's been days where we have texted all day, playful banter and even
sometimes sexual just for her to be ice cold as you put it the second she
walks through the door. Like wtf happened in 2 hrs. The cold side eyes.
The pursed lips holding back toxicity.

Just start documenting everything. Record the interactions if you are in a
legal state to do so. Do not let her know you are recording though. Good
luck sir.

alllmostcool
Man, you said it perfectly. The playful texts but then ice cold angry
person the second home. That was such a mind fuck for me. Jekyll and
Hide is 1000% real

Phew-ThatWasClose
Whelp, it *is* her hormones so yes, you might say that. And "18 more years
of purgatory" implies you have a newborn. Congratulations!! But also Post
Partum?? May be playing a role? And there are some shades of
Narcissism in there. The paranoia, the checking on your texts, isolating
you, making sure you don't tell anybody about your situation. I hope she
doesn't know your reddit username.

Her working theory is you just wait for luteal to be a raging asshole every
cycle so you can try to blame her hormones? and then what? You'll
convince her she has a *treatable* disorder and Ashton Kutcher will jump
out from behind a door somewhere. Worst episode of Punk'd ever.

Nothing changes if nothing changes. 18 years of purgatory or try
something different. Something is going on. The best way to figure out
what is to pursue a diagnosis (p.18). If she won't then you can at least
download the symptom trackers (p.299) and get started yourself. If she
doesn't like it hand her a stack and she can track you.

The best thing to do about the fighting is <u>don't be there</u> (p.107) for it. It's <u>abuse</u> (p.211) and it's not okay. Greyrocking is a survival strategy not a lifestyle choice. Science has shown the best way to deal with anger, anybodies anger, is to take a time out. Greyrock only as long as it takes you to leave. Just half an hour, long enough for the Pre-Frontal Cortex to come back on line. Then you don't hear it and you'll recover faster.

But more importantly she doesn't say it. Saying things out loud is reinforcing because of multiple modalities. She thought it, she said it, and she heard it. Her brain takes all that in and thinks "she should know". Without you there to yell at she won't say it and she won't have to regret it, or rationalize it, later. So take break as soon as your neuroception tells you things are about to go off the rails.

Of course tell her you're going to be doing that. If it's PMDD then you have the opportunity to chat during follicular. Maybe it's not her hormones, but something is creating this tension every cycle and everyone will be better off if you <u>make a plan</u> (p.58). A big part of that plan is taking a break when things get tense.

But also <u>protect yourself and your kids</u> (p.56). She cornered you, got in your face, and kicked you out of the house in front of the kids. That is pretty extreme already and PMDD gets worse over time. If you hadn't left when she demanded it would things have escalated? And are the kids safe once you leave?

As hempknight said document everything. Just write up what happened and email yourself so it's timestamped and in the cloud. Record if you can, though that's a bit sketchy. Save your texts to the cloud (there are apps) so you have that record. But most of all talk to a lawyer about what an emergency situation might look like. When things get worse what do you need in place to quickly get the kids to safety?

Make no mistake. Unless she acknowledges there is an issue, seeks a diagnosis, and seeks treatment of some kind, things will get completely unhinged. Be ready.

Sorry to be such a bummer. :^{

> Old_Structure_856
> Agreed with above…you give facts in a very direct way…but some of us need to hear it that way

> Hillside_herder

Damn. yes the hot and ice cold is so hard

I have a small child too, it's tough.

Ultimately I have decided to leave if she won't change. It's more trauma
for the kid if I stay and she won't change. Slept in a motel room tonight.

> funkcatbrown
> Gosh. I was just telling a friend about the times I went to a hotel to get
> away and let her be alone with her own shit or because I was kicked
> out. We split a while back. I do not miss that shit at all.

McRotor March 9, 2025
The switch is so brutal. We have 2 kids under 10. Listening to how she
talks to them when in the 'zone' is heartbreaking. It's sounds as if she
does not like them or enjoy being with them. Tone of voice, attitude,
patience (zero), fun (also zero). She does stay 'professional' so not too
many rages. This is the complete opposite of her normal time when she's
loving and actively enjoys being with them.

Tough enough as the partner to feel actively disliked during the zone - but
at least we know why it's happening and that it's not "us" (despite being
told constantly that it is 100% "us"). I am fearful of the impact that it will
have on children.

Rollercoaster does not describe it. More like living with 2 entirely different
people each month.

PrestigiousEdge3719 March 30, 2025
I love it when they play the victim by claiming that you blame everything
on their hormones, when yes, it really is due to said hormones. : / Their
truth-seeker traits completely dissappear during the 2 weeks before the
period. They just act like children who need to be lied to in order for them
to be able to regulate their own emotions. Run like hell if you can get
away. And I recommend never marrying, as PMDD can show up in any
relationship suddenly and now you're stuck with a nightmare. Don't
marry, don't ever move in together, don't share bank/credit accounts.
Always have a foot out the door ready to flee incase the woman you're
with suddenly gets mood disorders due to PMDD or Perimenopause
(especially in middle age). IDGAF if this seems insensitive. Save
yourselves

The original post on the sub.[14]

---

14 https://www.reddit.com/r/PMDDpartners/comments/1izjx6s

Confused

Extension-Message-12 - September 13, 2025

I'm looking for some outside perspective because I feel stuck in confusion.

I've been married since 2008, we have 2 kids (15 & 8). My wife has PMDD, and life with her swings between the kindest, most loving person you could meet and raging conflict that leaves me feeling broken. The cycle has been years of yelling, blame, and name-calling, followed by calm and promises to do better.

I love my kids deeply and want to protect them, but I feel torn. Being home means being near them, but also stuck in a toxic cycle. Being away feels sad and lonely, but calmer. One psychologist told me I only want to go home for the kids, not for her, and that hit me hard.

I don't know if I'm overreacting, abandoning, or finally protecting myself. How do you know when you've reached the truth?

> Superb_Pie_8560
> You're being tortured by your wife's erratic behaviour.
>
> You clearly just want things to work for the sake of all of you but especially for your kids.
>
> I say this because I endured years of it myself.
>
> In the end, this will come down to how great your resolve is and how much emotional abuse/turmoil that you can absorb before too much resentment builds inside of you.
>
> I gave up and am currently going through a divorce. I'm sad, broken for my children, I feel betrayed by my wife and angry at what I have been made out to be but am not.
>
> I have also begun dating and am realising what normal is and how life could be so I'm very optimistic about the future. A life away from my every breath being scrutinised is worth the temporary feelings of emptiness that I'm currently going through.
>
> I wish you well and hope both you and your wife can make it through this horrible affliction.

Extension-Message-12 OP
I totally understand the pain you've endured, it hurts to be apart but hurts to be together. My resentment has slowly built over time, I'm always the one that's in the wrong, ok I'll do better, I'll go to more therapy. But I'm at the stage where it feels why do I bother anymore

Superb_Pie_8560
PMDD is a very difficult illness to live with both as a sufferer and as a partner.

My wife began smearing me to anyone that would listen and abandoned me and the kids most weekends in the end and that was where I reached my breaking point.

I hope for yours and your families sakes that you can all get through it 🙏

Extension-Message-12 OP
Thank you, not sure if I want to get through it with her anymore

Superb_Pie_8560
You're welcome.

I can completely understand that.

All I will say is that I'm realising that there is a whole new life outside of your current situation and despite a lot of my current feelings, that's one thing that has really given me the strength to carry on.

Only you will know your own situation though and my advice would be that if you feel like there's anything left worth fighting for, then don't give up!

Extension-Message-12 OP
Yes I understand, there's definitely a whole world out there waiting to be enjoyed. Sounds like you fought to the end and gave it everything, I know I'm so close to that point or maybe I'm there I just haven't realised yet. The close people I lean on for support every time this happens keep telling me to leave....

Superb_Pie_8560
I had the same. In the end even my own mother had

said that despite having kids, I had to call it a day. As I said, only you can make that decision but PMDD is a very long road and continues until menopause is over so ask yourself if you can live in this situation indefinitely and whether your mental health can take it. Mine couldn't.

Old_Structure_856
Agree 💯 with the ⬆️ …PMdd gets worse as they get older if nothing is done to improve the situation…and remember perimenopause comes before menopause and from my experience it exacerbates the symptoms. OP I wish you well, but understand the roller coaster ride that you will be on for in nothing changes.

Extension-Message-12 OP
The way I see it, it's another 10 years of this, more than I can handle

Extension-Message-12 OP
I don't blame you for not being able to take it, not many people could

Superb_Pie_8560
Thanks.

I did try, God knows I tried but in the end, I'd become a doormat for the sake of my kids and that wasn't who I am or wanted to be.

Strange-King8917
Same as this post. I haven't started dating but what I have been told is how fresh it is to know there are some really nicer potential partners out there.

SpecialistFirm5318
"A life away from my every breath being scrutinised is worth the temporary feelings of emptiness that I'm currently going through."

That hits the nail right on the head. I'm about two years out from divorce and can affirm. A life where you live under a scrutiny microscope is no life at all and the feeling of emptiness may be a lot more short-lived than you fear it will be.

steamedCreambun
I feel for you. Haven't been married as long as you, but we have a toddler. We are currently separated because she can't stand me right now. Honestly so effing frustrated. Been through the ups and downs time and time again and it's all falling on my shoulders. I'm desperate for stability and I just dont know if it's possible with her. Making a decision on this is so difficult with a child involved.

Extension-Message-12 OP
I totally understand your pain, you're damned if you and damned if you don't. I get left second guessing myself constantly, questioning whether I can do better, should I have done something different to avoid the current conflict!

Phew-ThatWasClose
Fundamentally PMDD is chemistry. Good intentions and will power will only get her so far. Is she diagnosed? If so the doctor should have told her about treatments. It's not good for the kids to be around that either. What is she doing about it?

Baking_Dude
Been married since 2006. Wife was diagnosed with pmdd in 2009 after it became hell on earth and made me regret my life choices. We have 2 kids (15 & 13) and for almost every day since their birth, my focus is them…not her. And certainly not me. I made it my mission to focus on the kids. Raise them right. Protect them. Shield them. Help them understand how to navigate the chaos when mommy wasn't feeling well. We spent a lot of time out of the house. Just the boys. And even though she said she didn't want to join us, I was an a-hole because I made sure the kids had a great day. After all these years, I'm realizing I need to take time for me. The boys are well versed in how to support mommy without causing any more challenges for her. I am in therapy…finally. C-ptsd. And it's a wake up call - how little care I applied to myself, because I martyred myself for the kids. I had to. I'm finally reconnecting with the me I used to be, doing little things that gave me joy years ago before I was suppressed for too long. Good luck, man. It's a long journey of soul searching and pain and a

lightbulb in the distance calling you to your true self.

Extension-Message-12 OP
Your story sounds so much like mine, do you have any regrets about
staying, or are you glad you did considering the toll it's taken on you? I
used to take the kids out a lot and now I've lost a lot of enthusiasm to
do anything from being beaten down so much, I'm at the end of my
tether

Extension-Message-12 OP
She tracks her cycle and journals about her feelings and that's about it

Still_In_It
I feel like I'm responding to a post I wrote. That's how similar PMDD
affects us. I have a son I've raised since he was 6 with her, her son. And
now I have with her a 6, snd 3 year old. They are the reasons I'm staying
with her for sure at the moment. I'm at the end of her monthly cycle now,
and it's my most depressing time in the world.

So you're not alone man. Trying to figure out what to do when you have a
Gizmo and a Gremlin on your hands at the same time. And I know that
sounds mean, but it's accurate. She's the nicest person to me in the
world, and then she says the meanest things she can think of, like you
said, name calling, trying to make me look bad to family and friends. She
doesn't know what she's done until it's over.

You absolutely are dealing with two different people. All I can say is, try
and do things together during the bad times like going for walks. Things
that she likes to do, and be very very busy with work and hobbies. Also,
hopefully she is on medication she needs. That's hard because when my
wife needs it the most, that's when she decides she doesn't need it and
says "where's your medication!?"

I know so many of these relationships end in divorce. I'm trying my
hardest. You are not alone dude.

Extension-Message-12 OP
Thank you for sharing your experience. Kids add a whole new
dynamic, I used to think I'll just hang on until the kids leave home and
then who knows, maybe I can be free. I'm at the point now where I've
been away for several nights after a minor thing turned into a full on
yelling frenzy at me for 6 hours before I thought I'm done. I'm starting

to realise I was only hanging on this long for the kids and them being exposed to this dynamic is not helping them.

Phew-ThatWasClose
That's when I left. When I realized I was not helping my kids by being there because I was shut out anyway, and it was actually hurting them (p.273) because they were learning all the wrong lessons watching us. Separate households with no fighting is better.

But also … 6 hours is way beyond insane. 5 minutes max. Tolerating abuse is not support. As soon as you realize it's one of *those* conversations … take a time out (p.107) You know from experience you're not going to talk her down or reason with her so just leave. She'll calm down a lot faster without you there because you are the lion (p.125). Then you can come back in half an hour, long enough for the PFC to come back on line, and don't talk about it until follicular.

In follicular talk about how to handle the next luteal. What you are doing now is not sustainable. Luteal is a lot more manageable, a lot less chaotic, if it's scripted. Try to create a plan (p.58) that meets everyone's needs. For her that may mean more rest, more distraction, isolating if need be. For you that means more chores, more taking care of the kids, and refusing to be being yelled at.

You can't do it for her and you can't do it by yourself. They're her kids too. If she refuses to even collaborate on a plan to lessen the conflict then it's time to find the exit (p.56). But document everything first and take the kids with you if you can. A diagnosed but untreated mental health condition is a big deal.

Extension-Message-12 OP
Watching the effect on the kids is the most painful part, I feel as a partner we just become numb after a while, at least for me anyway. If I take timeout I'm accused of stonewalling or not sitting with my feelings, so I end up sitting there enduring it for so long that I give up and go I don't care anymore and I don't know if I can care anymore, straw that broke the camels back. The challenging part for me is every time I leave the home for a few nights she's really nice and apologetic, I end up feeling bad, I return and the it's rinse and repeat. This time I'm not sure I'll return though, it's been 6 nights I've been away. I've asked for a 1 month trial separation and shared custody of the kids but she won't let the kids stay away with me and the only way I can see them is if I see them in the family home while she's in another room. I'm not

comfortable with being anywhere near her.

Phew-ThatWasClose
Yeah. The PMDD just wants to fight so it will twist up any excuse to keep you there. Accusing you of stonewalling when you're trying to take a time out is classic. Then order you to "sit with your feelings" while the PMDD yells at you. It's just manipulation and abuse.

For your own mental health do not comply. Six hours is ridiculous. 5 minutes to gather your things and head to the gym. She can call it whatever she wants but you are taking a time out. Adults have discussions, not six hour rage fests. She will calm down a lot faster if you're not there. Meanwhile the kids are learning all the wrong things. In my state spousal abuse while the kids are in the home is *legally* child abuse for that reason.

Document everything and talk to a bunch of lawyers (p.56). You don't have to do anything about it but you'll feel better knowing you have options. They're her kids too. She's okay with putting them through this every month? That is monstrous! You don't want shared custody - you want full custody.

The whole not letting you be near the kids unless she's in the next room - that's her pretending you are the abusive one, the untrustworthy one. She will tell the court about her "fears" and possibly make shit up. Ask the lawyer about that too.

SpecialistFirm5318
Can confirm the stuff about pretending you are abusive so that she can try to limit your time with your own children. Once she rings that imaginary bell, all it takes is one bad (or even disinterested) judge to realign the realities of your relationship with your kids.

Leaving was still the right choice by a long shot, but I'd be smarter about it if I had it to do over again.

Extension-Message-12 OP
I really appreciate your insight. The restriction that I can only see the boys if she's in the next room has been a big red flag for me too. I've started documenting these patterns and am discussing them with the mediator, and I'll be speaking with a

lawyer as well. Hearing your perspective helps me feel more prepared.

Extension-Message-12 OP
Thank you for this — it really rings true. The accusations of stonewalling and the hours of arguments are exactly what I've been experiencing. It's reassuring to hear I'm not overreacting by needing time out. I've started documenting and involving a mediator because the impact on the kids is becoming too much.

Phew-ThatWasClose
Excellent. A lot of us have been there so reach out of you need anything like advice, support, validation. It's a rough road ahead.. You got this!

The original post on the sub.[15]

---

15 https://www.reddit.com/r/PMDDpartners/comments/1ng76de

I have a question about this subreddit

Far-Structure-6933 - October 21, 2024

Why do so many people post about struggling with their partner abusing them, like beating them up and stuff? PMDD can often make people distant and emotional, but it doesn't not make people beat their loved ones up??

This post might get a lot of hate but I'm just really confused.

I stugge a lot with PMDD which often results in me doubting my (healthy) relationship. But i have NEVER had the feeling that i want to beat my partner up. I am aware that people experience PMDD differently, but that does not excuse literal abuse.

I also often see people commenting "that is not PMDD" on the posts I'm talking about.

I feel like many of the posts that are being posted here, should be posted on the relationship sub (or others like that) instead

HusbandofPMDD
It is true that most of the people here have relationships where there is abuse as part of the pmdd.

Not all pmdd sufferers are abusive towards others. It sounds like many direct these feelings of shame and anger towards themselves.

Those that have healthy coping mechanisms probably don't need to be here. I'm here less
and less the healthier my partner's behaviors become.

It is also true that abuse takes many forms, including verbal, emotional, and psychological.
If someone threatens their partner with words (threatening it ending in break up over trivial things), engage in love bombing (being distant in a way that your partner feels like they have to do everything to win your affection back), if you engage in darvo tactics, it's still abuse.

You're right, that PMDD doesn't make people abusive, but at the same time pmdd wouldn't be much except physical symptoms if there wasn't some kind of psychological interaction and some kind of emotional dysregulation.

Partners are people too. We are broken. Maybe we have a savior complex, maybe we faced our own trauma growing up. Maybe we stick around for those reasons, or our beliefs about keeping our word, or wanting what's best for our kids. Maybe we are holding on to hope that it'll get better.

This group exists to bring awareness of what pmdd can look like for the partners, give tools and tips for dealing with it, and provide solidarity for the broken and a space for them to unpack and heal.

There is a constant flow of new faces, as well as some old familiars. Some rightly disengage from an unhealthy, unchanging relationship, while others find information about treatment and nice forward with a happy life. Still more stick around and keep working on improving their relationships and are in the process of healing with their partner. Others become bitter and resentful. Still, the lobby is always full.

Count yourself happy that you win both the lottery of pmdd and the product of a stable, healthy upbringing... Or at least one that isn't negatively impacting your relationship. Don't be surprised that pmdd can get ugly, we're all human. Don't be worried that your puff doesn't look like someone else's pmdd.

Also, beware of the echo chamber of unhelpful validation that some pmdd groups offer. If you're only hearing, you're right, he's wrong, then proceed with caution.

TurbidArtifact
Also, as others have said elsewhere, this sub probably skews somewhat toward desperate folks struggling with the worst situations, and therefore features more abuse than PMDD relationships at large/overall. I feel like most everything I have read says the majority of relationships with PMDD partners do not feature abuse.

That said, IMHO, there are a lot of... interesting... sentiments regarding PMDD + abuse floating about on here, from both partners and sufferers, hence the previous commenter's suggestion to be aware of unhelpful validation, from all angles...!

EitherAccountant6736
I would say that 50% of the posts here are from partners trying to cope with the avoidant and abandonment side of things.

Trauma and surface in two forms (toxic shame and rage).

Phew-ThatWasClose
We get a lot of hate on the other sub because most women with PMDD do not abuse their partners and they cannot conceive how that could possibly be. Others think they would never do that so if someone did maybe there was a reason? Sort of the opposite of the more traditional blame the victim stuff.

Just yesterday a woman commented

There are a lot of ex partners and partners in that sub that will say any symptom of PMDD is "abuse." As a survivor of abuse, it's very infuriating to hear that.

I will say that as a survivor of abuse myself it is very infuriating to hear another survivor of abuse discount and invalidate my lived experience just because ??? Why? Because she has the same disorder my abuser has? So that means ... ? I think that means she's a *better person* than my abuser but then why is she ... invalidating ... and? ... WTF?

And truthfully we don't say that *any* symptom of PMDD is abuse. Just the abuse part. And even there we are extremely careful to point that out being abusive is **not** a symptom of PMDD, as you have noted.

Being abusive is a symptom of being an asshole. One possible symptom of PMDD is "Marked irritability or anger or increased interpersonal conflicts" If one has PMDD, and is also inclined toward assholery, the "increased interpersonal conflicts" may result in being abusive. PMDD doesn't cause abuse, but it does open the door. PMDD removes some of the guardrails that are otherwise in place.

Is like being an abusive alcoholic. Some alcoholics are the happy kind. Others, not so much. "I didn't mean it. I was drunk." gets old fast. If it's someone we love we can forgive, once or twice, but they damn sure better get that under control right quick. Unlike the alcoholic the woman with PMDD doesn't have the option of going to rehab and quitting PMDD. So some of us end up forgiving a lot more than we ought and staying a lot longer than we ought and really really suffering the consequences of that.

As H pointed out most women with PMDD have it managed and most of the rest do not experience rage as a symptom. Their partners are not here. Here we are the partners of the extreme cases that do experience rage as a symptom, don't have it managed, and, in some cases, don't give a shit. Disentangling all that is what drives this sub.

Good question. Thanks for asking. :)

> Far-Structure-6933 OP
> You actually gave me the answers i was seeking! The example about
> the alcoholic made it even more clear. Thank you!

The original post on the sub.[16]

---

16 https://www.reddit.com/r/PMDDpartners/comments/1g8s6iu

You Are Not Safe

In extreme cases PMDD episodes can go south quickly. Even if you stay in control and greyrock your heart out things can go awry and you will be blamed. If the police are ever involved the odds of you going to jail increase. If not that incident then the next or the one after that. Once the police are involved you are on the clock. Fix it or flee. Guess how I know.

These are some of the high drama posts. These are not the worst ones.

Abuse is abuse no matter the excuse.

If you wouldn't do it to a puppy don't do it to a human.

Tolerating abuse is not support.

It can't escalate if you're not there.

Greyrock as long as it takes to leave,
leave as quickly as possible.

As soon as you realize it is one of *those* conversations ...
Walk Away

Abuse is abuse is abuse

(Editors note: In the original post TG had all the info-graphics in a nice slideshow up top. Obviously we can't do that in a book so TG's post is followed by the nine infographics followed by members comments. Had to convert the graphics to greyscale for the book.

Also note TG did try to remove gendered pronouns but a few slipped through. Most abuse is Male->Female but obviously our situation is a bit different.

One member hijacked the conversation to say "it's more nuanced than that" and even though he agreed that *in this context* it mattered little he still felt a need to express his opinion *a lot*. I left it all.)

TasteGlittering4459 - January 15, 2025

Due to the societal view of men being unable to be victims of abuse, a lot of men are unaware of what abusive behavior actually is. Over my time observing posts here, I've seen so many textbook examples of emotional abuse being excused under PMDD. I wanted to share some resources I found useful when coming to terms with/exiting my abusive relationship, to hopefully help others do the same thing. One was needlessly gendered, so I edited it slightly.

You do not have to tolerate abusive behavior, even if it is caused by a mental health disorder. You're the only person in your life who is going to put you first, and this may be one of those times where you need to do that. The effects of abuse can be devastating. I left my narcissistic ex 7 years ago (was with him for 3 years) and I still get 'triggered' by stuff in regard to that relationship. If your partner is unwilling to take responsibility, the sooner you leave, the better for your mental health.

THE RELATIONSHIP SPECTRUM

Relationships can range from healthy to abusive, and some relationships may be unhealthy, but not abusive. Here's a breakdown of the relationship spectrum:

A Healthy Relationship	An Unhealthy Relationship	An Abusive Relationship
A healthy relationship means that both you and your partner are...	An unhealthy relationship starts when just one of you...	An abusive relationship starts when just one of you...
1) <u>Communicating</u> You talk openly about problems without shouting or yelling. You listen to one another, hear each other out, respect each other's opinions, and are willing to compromise. **2) <u>Respectful</u>** You value each other as you are. Culture, beliefs, opinions and boundaries are valued. You treat each other in a way that demonstrates the high esteem you hold for one another. **3) <u>Trusting</u>** You both trust each other, and the trust has been earned. **4) <u>Honest</u>** You are both honest with each other but can still choose to keep certain things private. For example, you both know that it is important to be honest about things that affect or involve the relationship and still know that it is also o.k. to keep certain things private. **5) <u>Equal</u>** You make decisions together and you hold each other to the same standards. **6) <u>Enjoy Personal Space</u>** You both enjoy spending time apart and respect when one of you voices a need for space.	**1) <u>Not communicating</u>** Problems are not talked about at all. You don't listen to each other or try to compromise. **2) <u>Disrespectful</u>** One or both partners are inconsiderate toward the other. One or both partners don't treat each other in a way that shows they care. **3) <u>Not trusting</u>** There is suspicion that your partner is doing things behind your back, or your partner is suspicious of your loyalty without any reason. **4) <u>Dishonest</u>** One or both partners are telling lies to each other. **5) <u>Trying to take control</u>** One or both partners sees their desires or decisions as more important. One partner is or both partners are focused only on getting their own way. **6) <u>Feeling smothered or forgetting to spend time with others</u>** So much time is spent together that one partner is beginning to feel uncomfortable. Or sometimes both partners spend so much time together that they ignore friends, family or other things that used to be important to them.	**1) <u>Communicates abusively</u>** During disagreements there is screaming, cursing, or threatening, or these things happen even when there is no argument. A partner is demeaning or insulting toward the other. **2) <u>Is disrespectful through abuse</u>** A partner intentionally and continuously disregards your feelings and physical safety. **3) <u>Falsely accuses the other of flirting or cheating</u>** A partner suspects flirting or cheating without reason and accuses the other, often harming their partner verbally or physically as a result. **4) <u>Doesn't take responsibility for the abuse</u>** The violent or verbally abusive partner denies or minimizes their actions. They try to blame the other for the harm they're doing. **5) <u>Controls the other partner</u>** There is no equality in the relationship. What one partner says goes, and if the other partner tries to change this there is increased abuse. **6) <u>Isolates the other partner</u>** One partner controls where the other one goes, who the other partner sees and talks to. The other partner has no personal space and is often isolated from other people altogether.

<u>INSTRUCTIONS</u>: *Give an example from real life or make up a story about a couple in one of these relationships and include all 6 of the traits.*

ABUSE DEFINED:

IT IS NOT:

- **a lack of control**

  It's a system of values, attitudes, beliefs—ways of thinking.

- **a mental health problem**

  It's a way to disorient a victim into 'helping' the abuser, rather than setting boundaries.

- **a nice Person with an anger problem**

  It's a grooming process to convince a victim that they're safe, when they aren't

IT IS:

- **a thinking problem**

- **an integrity problem**

- **an empathy problem**

ABUSIVE BEHAVIORS ARE **GOAL-ORIENTED**

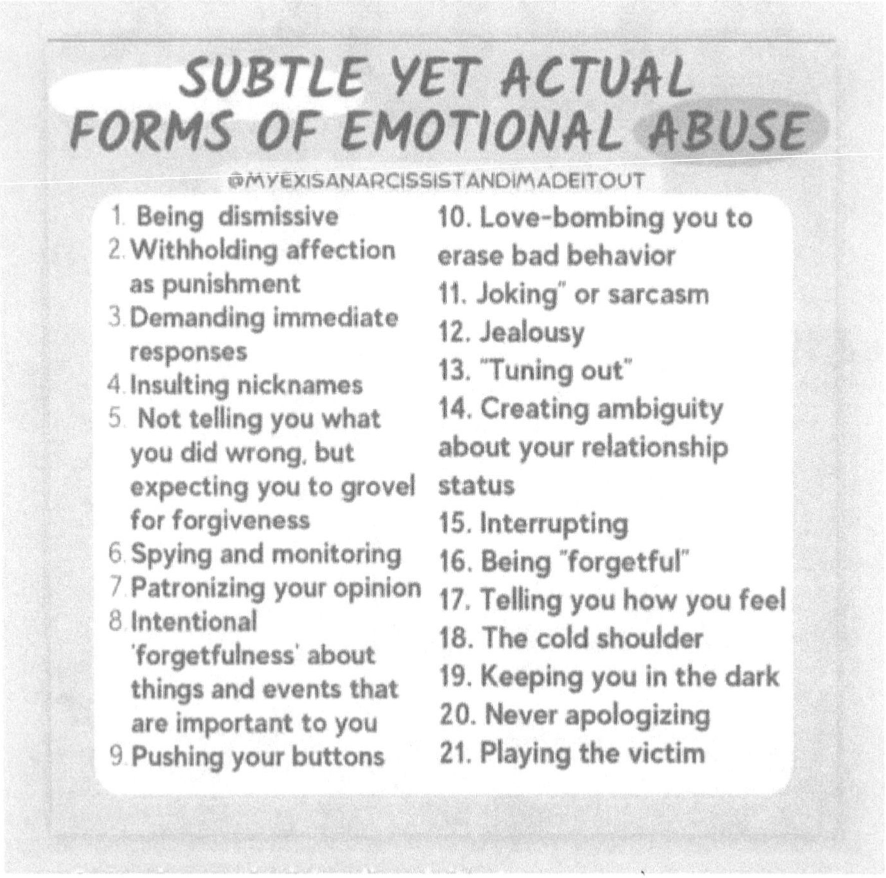

SUBTLE YET ACTUAL
FORMS OF EMOTIONAL ABUSE

@MYEXISANARCISSISTANDIMADEITOUT

1. Being dismissive
2. Withholding affection as punishment
3. Demanding immediate responses
4. Insulting nicknames
5. Not telling you what you did wrong, but expecting you to grovel for forgiveness
6. Spying and monitoring
7. Patronizing your opinion
8. Intentional 'forgetfulness' about things and events that are important to you
9. Pushing your buttons
10. Love-bombing you to erase bad behavior
11. "Joking" or sarcasm
12. Jealousy
13. "Tuning out"
14. Creating ambiguity about your relationship status
15. Interrupting
16. Being "forgetful"
17. Telling you how you feel
18. The cold shoulder
19. Keeping you in the dark
20. Never apologizing
21. Playing the victim

7 signs of covert abuse:

- Patterns of 'low-level' disrespectful behaviours, such as criticising, demeaning or undermining you.
- Less frequent abusive outbursts which are viewed as 'out of character' or 'having a temper'.
- An undertone of pressure to comply in the relationship.
- Micromanaging how you behave, socialise, finances and the relationship, through guilt, rejection or punishment.
- When you bring up their behaviour, they deny, blame or twist your words.
- You are labelled crazy or oversensitive.
- Ignoring your boundaries because what they want is prioritised above all else.

@thepersonalgrowth.project

5 traits that underlie an abusive mindset:

Overly controlling behaviour - a need to control others, often through manipulation and aggression
Entitlement - feeling superior or victimised (or both) and deserving of special treatment whilst treating others with minimal regard
Self-centred attitudes - doing what's best for them without considering the needs of others, even if it causes harm
Rigid gender-role stereotyping - unrealistic and harmful expectations based on gender stereotyping
External locus of control - a belief others and their environment are the cause of their behaviour, leading them to shift responsibility, blame, and less likely to change

@thepersonalgrowth.project

REASONS COUPLES COUNSELING
ISN'T RECOMMENDED FOR ABUSIVE RELATIONSHIPS
1 The vast majority of counselors have little to no training in the dynamics of domestic abuse, whereby one partner seeks to control & subjugate their victim.
2 Lack of training can result in victims being diagnosed as being 'emotionally unbalanced', rather than the abuse being identified as the true cause of the emotional instability.
3 Misdiagnosis shifts blame toward the victim & amplifies the abuse, rather than addressing the cause - the perpetrator of the abuse.
4 Many are trained in 'there are always two sides to a story', each partner must take 50% of the responsibility. There is no 50/50 responsibility when it comes to abuse.
5 Professionals may encourage victims to work towards 'saving the relationship', thus unwittingly placing the victim in grave danger.
6 Lack of experience results in the inability to see through the 'charm offensive' used by partners with sociopathic, narcissistic or psychopathic disorders.
7 Overwhelmingly, counselors, psychologists & psychiatrists have minimal training in the dangers of anti-social personality disorders.
8 Without an understanding of anti-social personality disorders, professionals may succumb to perpetrators manipulation tactics.

Abusive Behavior	Human Behavior
Loses their temper, then blames you for it.	Loses their temper, then apologizes and repairs.
Gives advice and demands that you follow it or risk punishment.	Gives advice but empowers you to make your own decision.
Blames all mistakes on you or someone else.	Makes a mistake and takes ownership for it.
Lies in order to make you feel crazy.	Lies and then seeks forgiveness with humility.
Says mean things in order to hurt or make you doubt yourself.	Sometimes says the wrong thing, but actions consistently show care.

www.alisoncookphd.com

HOW TO KNOW IF AN ABUSER IS CHANGING 1/2

1. Admits to ALL abusive behavior, past and present

2. Acknowledges that the abuse was wrong

3. Acknowledges that the abuse was HIS choice

4. Recognizes the pain he has caused and shows empathy

5. Identifies beliefs and values that led to his abusive behavior

6. Replaces abusive behaviors with safe respectful behaviors

7. Replaces distorted views with positive empathic views

8. Gives up double standards and entitled attitudes   @btr.org_

9. Is accountable for past and present actions by fully accepting the consequences of those actions

10. Commits to and honors making restitution and a living amends to his victims

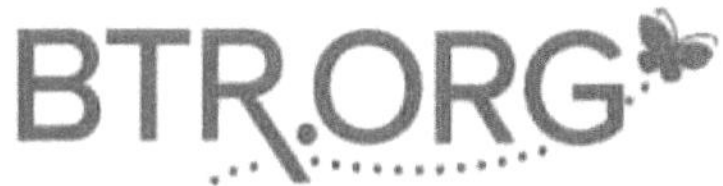

5 PARTS OF A SAFETY PLAN

The most dangerous time for someone in an abusive situation is often when they attempt to leave. **Safety planning is crucial.** A safety plan can be created before obtaining a protective order. Be kind and patient with your friend and remember that they are the expert on their own situation. Use these tips below to talk through a safety plan with your friend.

OVERNIGHT ESSENTIALS

Pack an **emergency overnight bag** for you and any children.

Give it to a **trusted** friend or family member to keep for you. Include extra car or house keys, diapers, toiletries and medications.

INTERNET/SOCIAL MEDIA

Be aware that your internet use **may be monitored** and take precautions accordingly.

Store important digital information in a **password protected** file.

RECORD ABUSE

Identify a safe place you can keep track of the abusive behavior and incidents. Or ask a trusted friend to keep records for you.

Date each incident and describe what happened. Take photos if applicable.

DOCUMENTS/ MONEY

Copy and **gather important documents** in a safe place (financial account information, children's birth certificates, SS cards, etc.). If you are able, start putting cash away in a safe place.

Keep important phone numbers or emails on hand. These can include an attorney, a domestic violence advocate, a therapist, or your local women's shelter.

SAFETY

If there are weapons in the house, **know where they are** and think about how you might get rid of them.

Think about **escape routes** within your home. Imagine how you would utilize the space to keep yourself and your children safe.

Teach your children **how to call 911** or talk about which contact to call in a situation of danger. Plan a "code word" with a trusted friend who also knows your safety plan and knows what to do if you text or call with the "code word."

FIGHT AGAINST DOMESTIC VIOLENCE™

National Domestic Violence Hotline:

1-800-799-SAFE

TasteGlittering4459 OP
Looks like I forgot to edit the gender out of a different one (how to know if an abuser is changing). I sincerely apologize.

> **P4p3rC4t**
> That one is kind of wild. Like, what if HE was the VICTIM? is the abuse still HIS fault??
>
> But good on you for speaking up on this stuff! :3

Phew-ThatWasClose
OMG! Thank you for doing this. Without objection I'm going to link to this from the wiki.

> **TasteGlittering4459 OP**
> Go for it! :)

Total_Plankton_3830
My only issue with this is "jealousy" being listed under a subtle form of abuse. Jealousy is a human emotion. Obviously how we handle things

when we are feeling it count, but yeah.

AzurreDragon
I wish this wasn't gendered

Fine-Arachnid4686
I don't believe this type of material is helpful or educational. It lacks the depth, the context and the nuance to evaluate complicated human relations. I especially don't appreciate that the material argues against counseling, claiming therapists are not "trained" in abusive behavior, as if this was a branch of knowledge instead of a complex diagnosis of a relation based on a history, evidence and conversations.

I'm glad that you are out of an abusive relationship, and don't pretend to question your experience at all. At the same time, I don't believe terms such as abuse and narcissism should be trivialized and reduced to a rule-of-thumb checklist that is posted on Instagram.

TurbidArtifact
I don't think anyone saying this is the end-all-be-all sum of all knowledge on abuse. What it is is a lil' collection of things that might help an isolated, confused, unknowingly abused person start to realize what is going on in there relationship. Every little bit helps. Also, it's not arguing against counseling - it's arguing against COUPLES counseling, which is most-often (from what I've read) not recommended in abusive situations for the reasons stated, among others.

Fine-Arachnid4686
I know this is walking on thin ice given the gravity and risk of certain specific situations happening out there, but I honestly believe we have become obsessed with some of these terms that were used to describe very specific situations. And part of the reason is that many human behaviors can be framed as narcissistic or even as abusive if they are not understood in the context of relational dynamics. I want to underline that abuse exists and narcissism is a thing and entails complicated behaviors, but this kind of pop psychology that floods social media has trivialized the meaning of these terms to the point that everyone believes they can identify and diagnose narcissistic behavior and abuse, which is clearly not the case, and in a time where we have become increasingly isolated, individualistic and self-centered, it is easy for people to misread conflict, which is inherent to any type of human relation, as abuse, abusive behavior, violence, toxicity, red flags and so on.

As for the couples counseling, I'd like to see more evidence and in depth analysis that shows how professional therapists are not in a position to determine when a relationship is abusive. I believe people who have the training and background and experience in couples counseling are much better positioned to identify these behaviors that most people, and definitely can provide more accurate tools, nuanced understanding and support than social media posts.

TasteGlittering4459 OP
The national DV hotline does not recommend you seek counseling with your abusive partner. Emotional abuse falls under domestic violence. Hope this helps.[1]

Fine-Arachnid4686
I totally understand the point. The issue is that a conflictive relationship might be labeled as abusive (many relationships fall in a grey area, as most of us in this group know). Again this does not mean that there are no instances of abuse where people feel forced to "work things out", instead of moving on and breaking with the abuser/abusive behavior.

My concern is that people become trapped in the idea that relationships can be conflict-free, jealousy-free, perfectly balanced, etc. We all, at different times, exhibit certain behaviors that can be labeled as narcissistic and even abusive. While I agree that it is important to have these labels, I don't believe they should be simplified because they are powerful and carry a specific weight in our society.

I wish I was more eloquent to make this point, but I hope this clarifies a little why I am wary of sharing media posts that convey very complex information in a very shallow format. I obviously would like for society to have more conversations about abuse, what it means and how to address it. I just wish it was in a much more meaningful way.

Phew-ThatWasClose
You may have a point about society writ large. Many "abusive" behaviors are just part of normal conflicts we all have. That was the thing that got me. Conflict isn't inherently wrong, but it's a matter of degree. Constant, unreasonable, manipulative, and

---

1   http://www.thehotline.org/resources/should-i-go-to-couples-therapy-with-my-abusive-partner

controlling conflict is abuse.

We are here. We are in *this* specific situation dealing with *this* specific disorder. Often PMDD isn't that bad in the beginning, or only shows up after childbirth, or can be masked by co-morbid conditions, for *years*. Often partners arrive here after having experienced slowly escalating abuse over a long period of time and it's like the frog in the pot. They can't quite identify what it is but it sure feels wrong.

That, and the abuse itself causes low self esteem, lack of confidence, and brain fog. Personally I was pretty sure it *wasn't* abuse because it was never physical. Moreover I was so exhausted and completely twisted round by the constant whiplash of doing as I was told and then that was also wrong that, as partners often describe, I was a shell. During the divorce I got dinged for being incompetent and irresponsible while *also* being accused of being threatening and domineering.

It wasn't until two years after the divorce, when it became clear I wasn't the problem, and she got the diagnosis and the help she needed, that I came here and slowly realized that yeah, that was years of abuse I went through.

So when partners arrive here still in the thick of it and say things like "oh, but it's a mood disorder so just have to be understanding and not take it personally." that's only partially correct. Like I said I thought it *wasn't* abuse because it wasn't physical. A pop psychology list/meme/info-graphic would've helped a lot if I had seen one earlier.

> Fine-Arachnid4686
> Thank you for articulating your experience into the discussion. I always find that is helpful in the context of this sub.
>
> I agree that these posts will be helpful for some people, like they would've been for you or for OP. My concern is that, for the majority, these might be reductive and lacking nuance. It is hard to question these things given that they are useful for people in very vulnerable situations. However, I think we live in a time when self victimization is a constant temptation. Self-help, which to me is the precursor of this kind of pop psy that is all over social media, pushes for extreme individuality and is not a pro-social current of thinking. I just want to point out the dangers of such approaches at a time when relationships are

under absolute scrutiny but antisocial behaviors and isolation are not. Outside of this sub, I've seen hundreds of lonely people complaining about failed and short lived relationships, incommunication with potential partners, frustration about "situationships" and orbiting and ghosting and so on. Part of this, I believe, is the reticence to accept conflict as a natural part of our interaction as human beings, and the unwillingness to work through problems with people with whom we want to build meaningful relationships.

Anyway, I understand why these should be visible for people on this sub. I would just say: they should be taken with a grain of salt.

Just my two cents.

TasteGlittering4459 OP
I agree that narcissism/npd has had an unhelpful reductive treatment on social media. However, that doesn't negate the usefulness of the term "narcissistic" to describe a pervasive pattern of selfish and self serving behavior. I do think terms such as "narcissistic abuse" do as you're saying and try to reduce complex human behavior down to a set "pattern".

The other comment replying to you is correct, it's not an end all, be all description of abuse. Rather, it's a small collection of signs that might help someone get out of the FOG that comes along with abuse. I included the image about couples counseling because I've seen more than one instance of couples being dismissed by their counselor in this forum. Those reasons listed may be a contributing reason why, which they seemed unaware.

I'm confused as to why an increased knowledge of abusive behavior isn't helpful? It is not oversimplifying human behavior to acknowledge some behaviors are abusive and a pervasive pattern of such is a sign of an abusive relationship.

friendly-ontario
Can the mods pin this? This is one of the most useful posts I've seen in a while and will help future members of this community.

miliefisathand

I met someone who was all 3 depending on the mood

Itchy_Ad_6713
Thank you.

The original post on the sub.[2]

---

2 https://www.reddit.com/r/PMDDpartners/comments/1i1vjav

Nobody understands, nobody is listening, it's driving me crazy.

(Heads-up: deals with abuse…)

TurbidArtifact – October 17, 2024

I recently realized, after having a mini mental breakdown of sorts, that I have been emotionally/verbally (and occasionally physically) abused for 10-15 years or longer. I brought up this abusive behavior with my partner around four months ago, and we've been working through this mess since. Though she admits there was definitely abusive behavior, that behavior has not totally stopped, either, and she has actually been hurtful/cruel *about the abuse*. She has PMDD, and *has* taken steps to address it - SSRI, therapy (individual and couples), etc.

Why I'm here is… I feel like nobody understands what I'm going through. I feel totally alone, unheard, adrift, invalidated.

I'm not close enough with my family to talk about it. I don't have close friends nearby, plus my wife shares those friends and I don't want to make it weird. My therapist - to his credit - does not just come out and say "You're being abused," he lets me come to my own conclusions (though, he did recently say, "It sounds like, from what you're telling me, that this is an abusive relationship.") Our couples therapist - again, to her credit - is giving us both equal time to share our hurt/issues, and isn't making any declarations either. And my partner has been (IMHO) dismissive and defensive about it more than she has been apologetic or understanding. She also shares with me *her* therapist's opinions, which seem to be… very sympathetic to *her* struggles over *mine*, let's say, which I understand to an extent (it's her therapist, after all.)

These issues are all compounded and complicated by PMDD being in the picture. Though my wife agrees PMDD does not necessarily *cause* or *excuse* abuse, she also still holds tight to the idea that the abuse would not - and will not - happen without the PMDD. To me, a contradiction, but… apparently not to her? She even seems to think I'm being too hard on *her* about the abuse, considering that she struggles with PMDD. (For example, we just had a conversation about me feeling unheard in all the ways listed above, and her response was, "Do you think it might be because it's not as black and white as you think it is?" I.E., because PMDD is in the picture, I'm not going to find the sort of validation I am seeking.) I don't know what to think about all of this. Her therapist (or at least what I hear through my wife) seems to think the behavior is normal for a PMDD sufferer and has even made comments that make it *sound like* the PMDD is a valid "explanation" for the abuse. My individual therapist and our couples therapist aren't PMDD experts, so they kind of don't really say much about it. My wife's family doesn't know about the abuse, but have recently heard more about her struggles with PMDD, so they're really sympathetic with her at the moment, which I also get.

Now… I know I'm really just seeking validation right now, and also know that validation is of questionable value; I need to come to my own truth. But it's so hard to do that! My mind is already crumbling, and I was shocked to find out I was being abused in the first place, so it's *still* difficult for me to admit or even believe solidly… and now everyone around me is either being as neutral as possible, or is actively trying to convince me I'm overreacting. It's literally driving me crazy. It's like I'm *screaming out* "HEY, I'M BEING ABUSED!?" and everyone's reaction is like… "Hmmmm, interesting." Or, "But… PMDD." It's so frustrating, and I worry this muted response is going to cause me to slip back into that initial state of uncertainty about the abuse. I can sense myself starting to go, "Well, if nobody is shocked by this behavior, and seems to be hesitant to just come out and say, "You're being abused, this is bad, something has to change"… I might start believing I AM overreacting, even though I've worked hard to get to a place where I (almost) know I'm not, and I might start feeling like I AM being too hard on her! I also - like any human in a similar situation - feel like there should be *some* kind of… consequences?… for treating someone like I've been treated, but there's just nothing - and if anything, there seems to be *sympathy for the abuser* because of the PMDD!

Do any of you feel the same way? How did you handle it? Thanks, and good luck out there, y'all!

udontbotheridontbe
Once I realised I was both being abused and reciprocating abuse I made one of the hardest decisions of my life. I left. And it's been over a year, I still haven't been able to bring myself to say a single word to her. I'm still in contact, via email, due to kids. And even that contact gives me panic attacks.

I am happier and more at peace than I have been in 10 years. I'm also clean and sober.

Abuse is abuse is abuse. That's what I tell myself. No matter the cause or reason. Abuse is abuse is abuse.

TurbidArtifact OP

If you don't mind me asking, how long did it take from when you realized you were being abused to when you left? What was that period like in between?

udontbotheridontbe
Probably a bit over a year. Once I'd heard the excuse "because you pissed me off" one too many times, I said to her that's what abusers say. It only took weeks after that incident.

It was tense and both of us were unhappy. I ended up in hospital due to suicidal ideation, twice. The psych people had spoken to her the first time, it was promised to be better, fairer, less aggressive - it didn't change. I was blamed for my poor mental health. I was told my suicidality was put on, was to hurt her, was the reason she would "get pissed off" with me.

After the second time I never went back.

TurbidArtifact OP
Oh man. :(So sorry to hear that, but thanks for sharing.

udontbotheridontbe
Just do your best to stay true to who you are. Once I realised I was becoming someone I didn't want to be I knew it was time to change/leave. I hope you can work through your situation.

I was demonized to mutual friends before and after I left. She had told everyone I was on meth to explain my 'erratic behaviour'. I hadn't done meth in 3 years, 4 now. I don't have any friends left. I have a new partner who is like day to my ex's night. Life gets better and life will put you where you need to be

iloveherbuticant
Same and I was put on a 5150 hold. And guess what?!?! That is new material for her when she rages to be thrown in my face. "I don't have an issue but you are mentally unstable. I wasn't the one taken to the hospital and put on a 5150 hold"

Phew-ThatWasClose
I was diagnosed with depression and just that was thrown in my face and used for leverage. I had the mental health diagnosis, she didn't. She would divorce me and take the kids. Eventually she did.

Phew-ThatWasClose
Holy Fuck Buckets YES!!!

You are completely valid and legit to feel that way and hold firm and solid to that. YES it is abuse! YES it is wrong wrong wrong. NO PMDD is not an excuse or an explanation or a justification. YES you are owed a big ass apology and free beer for the *next* fifteen years. Fuuuuuucking Hell.

You've been gaslit three ways from sundown and Do Not Listen!!! Your eyes are open now. You are correct. Even if you're wrong you're right. You don't have to consider the other point of view. The other point of view abused you for over a decade. No. No. No. No. No.

I'll go calm down and maybe have something helpful to say later :)

Idioglossia101
So I am on this thread as someone who is a woman who has PMDD with a long term partner. I am on here for him because this allows me to see what other partners discuss or ask questions on and then I can go back to my partner and say "hi, how do you feel about this and this when I'm in PMDD, should we work on this together or is this something I need to work on?"

One thing I have noticed is that the community on Reddit of PMDD and in other spots, use PMDD as an excuse for their behavior. It's disgusting.

There was a point in my relationship (I can't fully remember now the context of this and what exactly happened) but my partner visibly did something and I had to stop and ask him oh my god am I being borderline abusive? How long has this building for? What's going on? In that particular moment I was in PMDD but still recognized it for what it was. We took a beat and said "let's talk when I'm out of PMDD" sure enough we had a long conversation when my period was over and I realized I needed to work on a few things. So I did that. The problem resolved and what we still struggle with we still work on with our couples therapist but never once has my boyfriend said to me "I'm feeling like this borderline behavior and I don't feel safe".

It sounds like even though she's willing to get help for her PMDD through SSRIs extra, she isn't self aware to understand how her behavior impacts others and instead continues to use this as a crutch. Point blank - this is not OK.

I think you need to take a step back and really look at your happiness, your needs, your love for this person and figure out if it's still worth continuing to fight.

Everything you are saying is valid. It's not okay.

While PMDD is something we cannot control and it fucking sucks, any mental illness or illness is no reason to allow yourself to treat others like shit.

I also want to recommend you find a men's abused support group and get some support in that way. Also IAMPMDD.org offers some webinar type groups for partners of PMDD. You may find some good help there too.

You are valid. You are a person who deserves love, safety and care. Please remember that.

Take care and goodluck!

SaltVictory8301
Bless your heart. This is such a great post. I relayed for years that I was being abused to her and there was zero accountability. I told her how low her words and actions were making me feel and was gaslit to make me feel I need to change and I'm a flawed person. I tried to set boundaries about verbal abuse, name calling, and rage but I was too beaten down to enforce them and she didn't care about what I had to say to her. My feelings didn't exist. There was only her and PMDD. Be very proud of yourself for taking a look at yourself, as well your partner's actions and working together to find common ground.

Idioglossia101
Thank you! I appreciate your kind words and I am so sorry you had to go through that. I hope you're in a much better situation now and with someone who loves you and cares for you like you deserve to be cared for and loved!

Phew-ThatWasClose
You are totally my hero right now!

Idioglossia101
Thank you for that comment, so kind of you! Honestly - part of the reason I am this way no is because of my mom. She has undiagnosed Borderline Personality Disorder and PMDD when I was

growing up. Seeing what she did to my dad made me realize that I can't do that to a person. My partner is a wonderful, caring and lovely soul. I would never want to break him like my mom did my dad (Although my father is far from perfect and had his faults too that caused my trauma haha). But yeah. I just wish more women with PMDD realized that accountability is part of the game. You can't just sit back and say "but I'm mentally I'll so it's not my fault" the world would be a much better place if we all took accountability - but that's alas a dream. So I do what I can instead :)

Phew-ThatWasClose

I had a similar experience with my therapist. He never came out and said "you're being abused". I wish he had. I get that therapists aren't "supposed to" tell you what's what but rather guide you to realize it on your own and "come to your own truth". But they have the training and the vocabulary. I didn't think it was abuse because it wasn't physical

I was sooo frustrated with what was going on and I kept trying to reason my way out of it and I just felt boxed in from all sides. I physically felt trapped and constrained, as if in a box. She told me I was doing it wrong and I "should" have done the other thing. So the next time I did the other thing and that was wrong because of … reasons. I couldn't "figure out" what I was supposed to do and it took years to realize I was straight up screwed no matter what.

We hate to think our partner, our love, our gem, is an abusive ass. We pay therapists to give us an educated knowledgeable third party perspective, not to just listen while we stumble around in the dark. It wasn't until I got here, four years after the divorce and a year after the diagnosis, that I even heard the word "greyrocking". I greyrocked for the last *two years* of my marriage as a last desperate attempt to just survive and had no idea it was a thing with a name, and a thing people did to survive *abuse.*

Vocabulary is empowering. Words like "emotional abuse" and "verbal abuse" and "reactive abuse". And other words like "gatekeeping" and "catastrophizing" and "hypervigilance". I was in it for over a decade with no words to describe my experience. To his credit my therapist did suggest, once, that I might have PTSD. I thought that was ridiculous, because I've never been in the military, and he let it drop. He could have explained about C-PTSD and trauma and the effect of long-term abuse, but he didn't.

I'm just now realizing that those episodes I've been calling "panic attacks"

- those are fucking flashbacks.

My sister attends Narcotics Anonymous which is a 12-step program for drug addicts. She says she feels like a second class citizen because everybody there has harrowing tales of heroin or cocaine or oxycontin or meth. She's there because she was addicted to pot, which isn't even addictive. I feel the same way when I lurk the cptsd sub. Those folks have such awful histories and are truly struggling to recover. And what happened to me? My wife was mean.

But abuse is abuse and trauma is trauma and it's not somehow made better by the fact that it could have been worse. Now your eyes are open you can extricate yourself. Sounds like you're doing it methodically, which is good. Take it slow but don't abide the gaslighting. Document everything. Most lawyers will give you a one hour consult for free. Talk to five and ask them what you need to document. I did not do that and she took the kids.

Maternal bias is real. Get a male lawyer. Divorce tends to be dominated by women. If you have a choice get a male judge. We did arbitration so we did have a choice. Our female arbiter could not conceive of a wife abusing a husband. When I told her I was not allowed to take the kids to the store she asked what I meant by "not allowed". In the end she dismissed my entire lived experience by finding me "not credible" and gave my wife more than she asked for. Similarly the PRE blamed me for my ex's gatekeeping. She said I needed to learn how to "make space" for myself if I was going to achieve my parenting goals.

I found couples counseling to be useless precisely because they try to be balanced. They mainly focus on better communication skills but when the power dynamic is completely one sided communication is all one way and "skills" are not the issue. And her therapist? You only hear what she says her therapist says and her therapist only hears her side. Don't take any of that seriously.

Another vocabulary word I cling to is "False equivalence" Is like both-siderism where yes, both sides do it, but one side does it 1000x more. It's not the same. I'm sure at some point in the last 15 years you did something that was not awesome. And I'm sure people are telling you you have to "own your part" and from there they slide easily into "both sides have some responsibility" and … suddenly it's 50/50. Don't fall for it.

That's what I meant in my earlier rant when I said "even when you're wrong you're right". Nobody is perfect but that does not mean you are "partially responsible" for your own abuse. Your abuser is 100%

responsible. You did not "let" her. You did not "cause" it by "triggering" her. Maybe there are reasons she has a short fuse. She needs to own that and take steps to mitigate it. Obviously don't be an asshole yourself, but don't excuse others either. It takes two to tango but it only takes one to trap another person and abuse them until they react and then claim it takes two to tango.

If it's 99/1 say that out loud. If it's 99.999/0.001 say that. If they want you to "own your part" say "you first". If they want you to forgive *and forget* say "ask again in fifteen years." Obviously don't dwell. You're coming out of the shadow. Take a deep breath and turn your face to the sun. Spread your arms wide and listen to the breeze. There's a road ahead and in the distance there is peace.

Happy to chat if you want.

TurbidArtifact OP
The part about "False Equivalence" really hits close to home for me. I've dealt with a lot of that, IMHO (including within couples therapy), and it's maddening… until you realize it's going on, then it's a bit easier to handle.

An example: she was being cruel *about the abuse* recently, and I let my emotions get the best of me and said "F*ck you, you're being an asshole!" That's literally the start and end of it - I walked away after. Also keep in mind, I probably swear at her like… two or three times a *year*, out of frustration… and she had been talking to me *way, waaay* worse than this, regularly, for 10+ years. Her response, via text, was this:

Pathetic.

Hahaha. I don't appreciate how you just verbally abused me. Now it's documented. You will talk to me however you want. Cool, abuser.

Yikes. How does it feel to be verbally abusive? Shit. It's wasn't the first time, but now that it's properly documented, you can't deny it. Don't get mad at me, Google says it's true and you love the Google. (My note: This is referencing the fact that I learned about what verbal abuse is by Googling it and realizing we ticked like all the boxes…)

It's funny as I am working on myself and making progress, you are getting worse. You are meaner, have way less control, and say really hurtful shit…like before I left, not caring about me being suicidal (My note: this was wayyyyyy misconstrued and twisted out of context). Say what you want, it was meant that way. You think it's you not putting up with stuff, which is funny. You can have boundaries and stick up for yourself without being a dick or abusive.

And now, when things are the hardest, you steep low. Total lack of control. You think talking to me however you want is going to make things better? That's how you treat people? Cool, very mature. I will tell YOU right now, that won't be happening. Don't let the door hit you. If it's not about you, it's not valid these days. No, it's not your responsibility to help me, but it is your responsibility to try and not be mean. That's how I know YOU don't understand. You wouldn't be this way if you did. I'm good, I don't need you or expect you to do anything.

I must say, though, you keep saying you have to figure out if you can be with me and on and on. Jokes on you, I am figuring that out, too. Haha, it's looking like I will be well on my way before you know what's up or down. I am sorry that my growth is a threat to you. That sucks and says a lot about the work you have to do on yourself. I'll be happy to celebrate your growth. Why? Because I like to see you happy and succeed. When I'm down, I don't need you to stop making growth. I like seeing you well. It makes me happy.

Toodeloo!

Makes me sad to reread this now. :(Maybe it doesn't come off as cutting to y'all as it does to me, because I know all the context, but… she's saying this to a *person she has abused*, who is still *very hurt and angry and figuring it all out!*

(And, there has not been any message of this length addressing/apologizing for *her* actually-abusive behavior, either!)

> Phew-ThatWasClose
> Yeah. That makes my stomach churn. A lot of us have been there. My ex accused me of abuse and worse. She used to say the most vile garbage but she never yelled. Then if I yelled I was "intimidating" and "coercive". Because I'm the male I'm stronger and therefore scary. Somehow the fact that I asked her to stop 5, 10, 20 times first never mattered much. One time, just to see what would happen, I asked politely 100 times. Then I pointed out that I had just asked her to stop 100 times. And she kept on.
>
> Document this. Write up what happened and why you swore. This

reads like a desperate attempt to not take responsibility. If you hadn't said what you said it would have been something else. My ex used to say my demeanor was threatening or I had wild eyes or "she could tell." Like with the suicide stuff, she'll take anything and twist it, so don't let her convince you swearing is a bridge too far.

Do write it down though. She was cruel about the abuse. What did she say, exactly. Did she say you deserved it? Did she say you let her? Did she say you triggered her? Did she say you're too sensitive and quit whining? Did she say a real man would've … something? Write it down as objectively as you can and as much of the last 15 years as you can stomach.

You're never going to get an apology. You're trying to figure it out for you. You don't need her input. She's done enough. Somewhere along the way you lost yourself. That's what you're trying to find. Remember who you were 15 years ago? That guy!

And next time walk away *before* you say the thing. It'll drive her crazy.

> TurbidArtifact OP
> I write everything down now.

udontbotheridontbe
Reading that hurt. It so closely mirrors my own experience and could've been written by my ex. I'm not going to reopen and post those texts but my god, it gave me a chill to read it. I hear you man, you are not overreacting.

straightchaotic
These are the words of a sociopath. She was baiting you. You are not to blame. You are better than her and this.

chillpill
This hits so close to home. The reactive abuse. Gaslighting. Baiting. Suicidal ideation. Reading your post, I can relate to it 100% and you are not alone. I'm in nearly an identical situation as you. But I will say when my partner started doing work on herself, the physical abuse (slapping, spitting, hitting, throwing objects) has mostly stopped. But what remains is the verbal abuse, belittling, and constant gaslighting. I will say, I've learned to take none of it personally (although that's near impossible) and hear EVERY one of her gripes about me as a

gripe about herself. Chances are your partner's self esteem is very low, and takes that vulnerability out on you. But turning her insults around (I do this in my head while grayrocking) I can get through it. When she says "you're an awful father, only think about yourself, and am a threat to this family" she's really saying "I'm an awful mother, only think about myself, and am a threat to this family." I wish you luck, and know you can get through this. I'm still dealing with similar issues every month, so hoping we both come out of this stronger.

> TurbidArtifact OP
> Thanks for sharing! That's pretty incredible that you're able to do those mental gymnastics. Like you say, though, "it's near impossible" to truly weather that kind of storm, so... just be careful that it doesn't take more of a toll on you than you realize.
>
> I didn't *think* I was taking any of the abusive talk that seriously or personally... then all of a sudden one day, BOOM, my mind kinda' crumbled, in the form of semi-depression, anxiety, and a scary loss of ALL self esteem. E.g., "Does everyone secretly hate me because I'm a fucking loser?" "Am I a disgusting person?" "Do I even have normal interactions with other humans?," etc. It didn't make any sense, until I read the effects of long term verbal abuse, and it's almost textbook.
>
> All along, it seemed like the big blowout fights with physical stuff and the really heinous verbal abuse were the problem... but in hindsight, I think it was the constant drumbeat of little digs and insults and gaslighting and manipulation that really did the most damage. I think you are in a slightly better positing since you *know* what is going on and are actively dealing with it, though!
>
> So... be careful, but best of luck in whatever path you choose!

> > chilllpill
> > Thanks the support. But what you said really hits home. It's like the abuse found a way to seep in. I wake up and hear the insults on repeat. And the constant digs, belittling, name calling. If you come up with any resources to help with this PTSD, let me know. And did SSRIs help at all with your partner?

> > > TurbidArtifact OP
> > > Yes, the SSRIs did help! The worst of the worst/physically abusive blow-ups did stop, for the most part, even with just a

very low dose. The verbal abuse did not stop, however.

chilllpill
I just started reading about narcissistic word salad. Does anything of this sound familiar to your situation?
https://abusewarrior.com/abuse/narcissistic-word-salad/

gorybones
Marijuana is extremely mentally addictive and causes mild physical withdrawal symptoms and a percentage of people who smoke are addicted - it's called marijuana use disorder.

Phew-ThatWasClose
Thanks.

straightchaotic
Nah! @gorybones doesn't deserve a sarcastic "thanks". I stan you, buddy

straightchaotic
Uhhh, ok, not needed here in a thread about abuse and being disregarded and minimized…. Read the room and get outta here

gorybones
Wow, maybe you read the room or seek some therapy if my simple little comment triggered you that bad lmfao, yikes. I was just correcting a huge misinformation lie in that persons post but okaaaaay yikes

nogeologyhere
I'm so glad I found this sub as I've had repeated experiences of pmdd-based abuse and situations that have led to being very scared. It's good to know what was going on and that I'm not alone

TurbidArtifact OP
Yeah, I was very hesitant to post here myself - partially because I know she keeps an eye on this sub and will probably make fun of me for posting (Burner account, but I'm too specific with details…) But, I did it because I do get some solace out of reading other people's

experiences, and was hoping putting my stuff out there might make someone else feel less crazy, too. :)

straightchaotic
This is the tip of the iceberg of shit, as I read your thread about her text, those are the words of a sociopath, PMDD or not… You need to leave her, straight up. Take the steps to separate your life and find a service for domestic abuse victims. Get out of there and away from your friends (which you say are really HER friends). They are her agents.

If you have friends from before her, reach out to reconnect. If you have friends in a hobby or community that is only yours not hers, dial up asking them to hang out. You can confide that you are going through some stuff and "need a distraction." Judge accordingly if it is best to open up and how much detail you would good into. You need to start rebuilding your life without her.

Move away if you can and go no contact. Get a new phone, delete your social, take steps to protect your vial info like your social security number, bank accounts, and credit cards. Prepare for her to come after you to harm you, seeing her words she will (nothing is more scornful than the hurt pride of a wounded narcissist).

Consider everyone and everything you both share corrupted and tainted by her. Cut and run ♥

That-Armadillo8128
It's not for everyone. It can be difficult to stay engaged but somehow create distance when you know what they're saying is being fueled by the PMDD *and* resist the urge to bring up everything when they're feeling well enough and grounded to discuss it *without* building up resentment. Again, not for everyone. So far though, I'm committed in my relationship and the overall good outweighs the overall bad to me, though yes it is the most difficult thing I've experienced.

TurbidArtifact OP
Yes, everybody has to make their own call. A couple's history, the particular flavor of their negative PMDD interactions, the effects those interactions have had on the partner's mind, the prospects for improvement… every murky mess is unique and requires a lot of work to figure out.

My anger is the issue?

JobAromatic7843 – July 2, 2025

Anyone else have their PMDD suffering partner accuse them of angry outburst when it's not anger? My wife is saying that she fears for her life due to my anger problems, but it only happens when we're in the luteal phase. For the record, I've never gotten physical in the slightest. I've never been physically aggressive in any way shape or form. Of course....she's trying to end our relationship now. She's told her parents (which make me look like the bad guy) and wants to tell the kids that we're separating. This time it's been going on for 4 straight days, though. She swears it's not the PMDD because she feels normal in every other way. This is also the first month of hormone replacement. She's on the estrogen patch. We're about a week out from her period.

ihaveredhaironmyhead
If she's threatening to break up with you just say ok and leave it be. Don't fight back against someone who's not rational. Just listen to what they are saying and calmly be yourself.

UpInWoodsDownonMind
You are definitely not alone my man. You need to remember that a lot of the time when they say things like this it is more of a self report than an accusation. Sometimes they will make you think that maybe you were too angry and sometimes maybe you actually did tell or raise your voice more than you wish you had. But they will take any frustration or push back you give them and call it anger because they know that's the easiest way to diver away from their own behaviour.

Write down some of your thoughts and wait until after her period has ended before trying to have a conversation. Talk to a therapist if you can and talk to her about possible options for managing her pmdd.

Reasonable-Weird258
This is one of the reasons I began voice recordings on my phone… Not to prove to her that she is wrong, but to prove to the police in case she ever makes any official claims. Even when she is not in the phase (sorry, still learning the lingo), she believes what she experienced from that period. It leaves me having to regain trust that is seemingly impossible to keep. Good luck, CYA. As another person stated, you can't discuss with someone who is irrational. You can bring up your concerns when she is

back… Hopefully your conversation goes better than mine.

Phew-ThatWasClose
In the moment perceptions are skewed. Anything, or nothing, can be perceived as whatever she needs it to be. "Reactive abuse" is when you rationally and justifiably defend yourself against the actual abuse and *that* is used as a reason for more abuse. If that makes any sense - it's like a triple negative or something.

Point is make sure it's nothing, and you can do that by not being there. Take a time out (p.107). It's frustrating as hell to not be able to defend yourself but you can't defend against crazy (p.54). Just walk away. Greyrock until you can leave then be elsewhere for half an hour. Long enough for the PFC to comeback on line.

Especially if she says she fears for her life. *You are not safe* at that point. That should be an immediate signal to walk. Hands up, back away slowly, grab your keys and out the door. Go get a froyo, hit the gym, find some nature and look for awe, whatever - but GTFO. Things can go south quickly and if the cops come someone (you) is going to jail.

The number one rule of PMDD is: No talking about anything substantive during luteal. Including luteal. And definitely including The Relationship. Next follicular talk about what went wrong this time and make a plan (p.58) to prevent a repeat. Likely that plan should include a lot more alone time for everyone. For now bring her tea, a blanket, and the remote. Then go clean the kitchen.

> JobAromatic7843 OP
> But she's been stuck in this for 4 days almost without relief…. It's not a half an hour and done situation.

> Phew-ThatWasClose
> Take some "you time" to clear your cortisol anyways. And greyrock like a mofo. Even walking to the other room and closing the door (p.125). If she has to trail you about the house maybe she'll have an awakening. *Ask* for a break. She's diagnosed. She knows it's luteal. "Even if it's not PMDD can we wait till next week to talk about this anyway?" or "My head is swimming and I need to take a break." Ask her to write down her concerns so she doesn't forget.
>
> Always low and slow. Consciously lower the speed and timbre of your voice. Have a seat so you're not taller than her. Move slowly. Pretend she's a scared puppy. Try a cold plunge to reset your

system if you feel the need. Pay attention to your <u>signals of anger</u> (p.114) and take that time out *for yourself* before you get activated.

Idk - try everything short of actually discussing it. Discussions go nowhere, never end, and can spiral out of control quickly. Words have power and the more she says it out loud the more true it becomes. Acknowledge and deflect. It's going to be a rough week. :<(

tx_hempknight
4 days is easy time. I get it up to 2 weeks. Take phews advice and walk away. This advice has been a godsend for me. You already know she's being irrational, so your big plan is to stay there and keep arguing? To be in her line of sight to continue blaming you for how she's feeling?

There's never going to be a moment of clarity for her where she snaps out of it and says, you know what, he's right. It's not going to happen. Go do something else. Throw her her favorite snacks and go into hiding for a while. Find some hobbies to pass your time until it blows over. I know it sucks, I know it's not what you signed up for. I know it's not how you want to live your life. I know this because it's how all of us feel about it.

Try getting her to do a vitamin deficiency test and see if she is deficient in anything. My wife was deficient in magnesium. With this I was able to convince her to take it along with a couple of other supplements that have shown to help alleviate it. She still gets moody and has outbursts but the last couple of months have been relatively mild and we have been able to talk and be around each other. But if it gets bad again, I will walk away. No point in both of us being overly stressed and fighting, she can fight by herself without me standing there.

Good luck brother and do everything you can to stay out of jail. What the PMDD mind thinks becomes reality and her reality can lead you into legal trouble.

redskrot
4 days would be heaven. I endure 2 weeks of hell per month.
I have always interpreted the anger accusement as some kind of projection or a validation for her to keep up her abuse.
Like if she pushes me to show the least amount of anger, i

immediately is the bad guy and it's for sure me who is angry and not her.

And if i, in her world, treat her badly she is in the right to punishing me.

No idea what goes on in her head for real though.

PadreDeBlas
3rd paragraph is textbook:

Especially if she says she fears for her life. You are not safe at that point!!!

Go get a froyo indeed! Because guess what, there's no froyo in jail. The quickest and easiest way for her to win whatever argument you're dumb/unlucky enough to be in is to bring the cops to your house. You know they don't leave empty handed on a DV call, somebody's going to county and it's probably (insert statistic too lazy) going to be you. Then you're fucked, especially with kids.

Love you Phew! Man, you always say it best, thank you.

Phew-ThatWasClose
Miss you around here. Hope you are doing well! :)

IbanArab
I'm in the same boat. Exact same. Calls her mom and tells her im abusing her again. Never laid a finger on her. I know verbally abuse counts but we're both doing that. My biggest mistakes are fighting back verbally and allowing myself to get angry (the same way she does). Shes 1 year postpartum so that probably doesn't help. My new plan is to:

- document her moods and behaviors to make sure its pmdd
- get therapy for me (years of this have messed me up)
- absolutely do not engage and get pulled into more unhealthy fights
- identify high risk times of the month and either evade or stay at a friend's house until she also takes accountability and gets help.

My friend's wife has pmdd and they've both been getting therapy for the last 2 years. He said they'd have 4 hours fights monthly and now rarely fight at all. There's hope if there's accountability. Good luck gentlemen

PolarBear1997
Stay strong brother

JobAromatic7843 OP
I'm so glad I found this group. You guys are saving my relationship.
Thank you.

HusbandofPMDD
Not that I'd call her bluff, but definitely state that these false accusations
are going to have a significant impact on your relationship. Have you
pointed this out to her? I had to honestly encourage my wife that if it really
was as she said then she should act or ask me to leave. otherwise I
expected those words to stop

Baking_Dude
All the freaking time. Any comment or question or insight is taken as an
insult or unsupportive or as though I don't care. I learned to say nothing.
Not a word. No reaction whatsoever. It took the wind out of her sails.
(Only recently learned the term 'grey rocking'). Unfortunately, I'm realizing
that, by taking it all in, I've carried too much for too long. If she wants to
leave, say nothing, let her leave. Put the onus on her to make the move
without you adding fuel to her fire. (Though be prepared, doing nothing
will piss her off too…you cannot win.)

Specific-Rest1631
Yes, it has a name, "reactive abuse"

Rothum90
My wife. Exactly my soon to be ex. All the anger issues were mine. I
definitely would lose my shit after 7-10 days of cruelty from her towards
me.

Naive-Weight-8766
7-10 days?! Good lord man. I thought I had it bad. Sorry to hear it…
hope you find peace of the other side brother!

Dry_War_747

> I have dealt with this exact thing nonstop, and have told her many times that I'm tired of being the "bad guy".

The original post on the sub.[3]

---

3   https://www.reddit.com/r/PMDDpartners/comments/1lqfij2

I want to understand how normal this is.

My wife has PMDD. How often do you see these traits?

Tubular_Jeeves126 - June 15, 2025

I have 2 jobs. Essentially 3. I am running two science publications, and one business one. I am exhausted, 24/7. I also am a very active parent to our child. Of the last 4 weekends, I took our son for a day with me (toddler) so she can feel better, as her moods were very bad.

I cook a similar amount to her. I pay all household bills. She is a school teacher. She does do pickups on the way home, I do not want to be unfair to her. Her main household responsibility is the food shopping. We have a cleaner as we both work.

So here's the list:

She is ALWAYS more tired than me. No matter what I've done, this will be true. When I come home with my son, I just get him in the house and put him to bed. If she does, it will ALWAYS be my job to unload his stuff, come out to the car, get him in to his bed, whatever. They do not arrive home without my involvement.

I have not seen a friend in 2025. Not since December 2024 socially. She has been out with friends 3 times in the last 2 weekends. She socialises regularly. That's fine, I'm happy she gets the opportunities. She typically has a VERY bad reaction if I am happy in my own company. She seems to need to fill time with constant distractions, buying things. Ticketed events. If I seem tired after my working week, and want a slow Sunday, that's usually going to be an argument.

When parenting my son, I am ALWAYS wrong. No matter how well founded, no matter how scientifically backed. I am wrong. We cannot have a discussion. She is generally offended if I put forward an alternative view.

I use a vape since our son was resuscitated. During COVID I was not allowed in the hospital building as it was one parent at a time. I started vaping as some sort of coping mechanism. I said I'd like to quit soon. She immediately gives me the "you won't be able to". I've never been a smoker, I am a gym guy, but my life is so relentless that it's become a crutch. I was not surprised by the anti-support.

I saved my son's life when he was having infantile spasms. Compared it with video evidence when the Dr dismissed it as sleep startles. He would have brain damage now if I didn't. I don't think I've ever been called a good dad, despite consistently having a lovely relationship with my son, and taking them both on big days out and holidays regularly (I literally drove them to Disneyland Paris from London, as an example). She will never let me feel proud as a dad, despite the fact we don't even have a dramatic lifestyle.

Out of the blue one day my son (4 with down syndrome), slaps his hand on my french bulldogs back. Not particularly hard. My wife says to me "did you just hit him?" (Meaning our son). Zero reason to suggest that, and she even knows me to be someone who literally can't even allow spiders and insects to be harmed. Yet she says that. Zero violence in our relationship, zero in my history, totally baseless.

I text her later saying "did you hit our son. Not great eh". She replies with "sorry I heard a sound". Never addresses it further.

On the subject of food shopping, sometimes when she has overspent on a night out, she just won't buy it. If there's enough for her and my son, she will just say to me "I had some toast." I'll come back home and the fridge has zero in it but butter. Regularly.

I respond by saying I might buy a meal prep service, so I can cope with the job and the parenting and the 5am wake-ups, as I've felt my body shutting down lately. She immediately responds with anger saying "oh great, what about us then. You're pulling away from US".

It is always US. She throws my son in to things. When she gets mad she does these othering statements, as if I am on the opposite side of the fence from him, despite the fact I have a lovely relationship with him, and spend most of the time playing with him, teaching him, building train sets and hot wheels tracks. These statements bother me immensely, but they just wash straight off of her.

She can make such strong statements, and then just not give a damn. Huge reactions to simple things like me wanting to be healthier, but when she says something really quite serious to me, it's nothing.

I did not know true negativity until being with her. I'm trying to deal with this all positively, and I do not want to split as I have really being trying to build a positive family, but PMDD seems to be more than just the week. There's a run up, a run down, and a complete absence of self awareness.

I have heard "you don't support me" so many times.
I have defended her from her mum "also had PMDD".

I have defended her in court and won. (Unjust parking fines)
I have paid all of her living expenses for a decade.
I have dropped her and been with her for any medical procedure.
I helped write her CV for her current job.
I have literally written school reports for her.
Trained her at the gym.
Saved our son's life and supported her enormously in a difficult pregnancy.

The strangest thing about all of this stuff is it seems she really doesn't like being without me.

To others, she tells them how smart I am. She tells them how I would never do the things some of the letdown husband's/boyfriends would do.

To me though? She tells me what I am not. What won't happen. How bad the future will be. How annoying my jokes are.

She also could say ANYTHING. I mean anything. She hears a term on things like Married at first sight, she will call me it. "Manipulator", "gaslighting". Whatever it is. Then takes it back immediately. If I seem disappointed in it, I go quiet. It's not worth the conversation as it will only escalate. The strange thing is, I tested it by basically acting like a saint. Didn't help. I'm avoidant now if anything. If she disagrees with me, there's always a risk I get called something pretty bad. It sticks with me though. Not her.

She then gets annoyed that it impacted me. I remember being told I was a bad dad, and then one day later it's father's way and I get a card saying "happy birthday daddy, thank you for everything you do for us". That was jarring. Awful feeling.

I really like myself a lot more on the days we are separate. Get on with everyone. Wish I could change it.

Phew-ThatWasClose
That's not normal. If there's no break during follicular it's not PMDD. Sounds like Borderline. PMDD often gets misdiagnosed as Borderline and vice-verse. If it's worse during luteal then maybe it's PME. Is she treating the PMDD? Or just using it as an excuse? As a friend of mine says "shitty people can be sick too."

Also - you are overstretched.

Tubular_Jeeves126OP
She's worse during PMDD yes. She's a good mum though. She's

lovely with my son in a lot of ways, as she uses all her teaching techniques, which is so valuable for DS.

She reacts badly when my behaviour doesn't align with what she wants. The thing is, I am very self aware, and I'd consider myself extremely strong. I won't agree just for an easy life. But I always make my points calmly. I've never dealt with something like this prior to her, never had a bad relationship.

I've just never seen something like this. Your days are fine with anyone else. Anyone. You encounter this person, and they will not allow you to be optimistic, they are always tired, always ill, always injured. Everything's always your fault. It certainly goes extreme that week, but it's like it doesn't switch off instantly.

Every now and then you get a period of respite, but it is relentless. I only work the 3 roles because she does not pay anything. I've expressed this to her a LOT. The problem is I do not want any escalation in front of my son (something that doesn't happen), and I do not want anger in my house. I am 40 now. 40 is supposed to be calm. There's something about the way she reacts that reminds me of reality TV.

> 97SPX
> Is she approaching or in her 40s? Hopefully you do know you're a good father and have done a lot for your family. You deserve a break and time away too. Nobody can keep giving constantly without a recharge.

>> Tubular_Jeeves126OP
>> She's 38, so yep. The bit that makes me feel very uncomfortable is I consider us to have a terrible dynamic now. We both wanted a sibling for our son with down syndrome, as I am a bit afraid of his future without it. He is the only one in his generation in my whole family (sister didn't have kids).
>>
>> We are low risk for down syndrome, and I'd want that, but tbh her behaviour is so awful, so often, that I am now finding that hard. When someone is this negative and able to switch so often, with so little accountability, what it kinda does it means that I cannot aim at anything in life with any true belief.
>>
>> She calls you whatever comes in to her mind, and then once a month simply says "I'm ovulating". That bit is sort of chilling. I feel cold.

97SPX
Perimenopause rocked my nervous system like nothing i had experienced before. Started before 40. But if there's no accountability outside of those moments its really hard to make any progress. The fatigue is crushing at times too, then add in hot flashes and insomnia. I wasn't prepared for this and didn't realize it for years as I was considered too young for Perimenopause. Hormone tests show that was incorrect, just missed. Good luck. Im saddened for so many navigating this all.

Tubular_Jeeves126OP
I forgot to mention, she has bought a range of supplements for the PMDD. She thinks she can feel me pulling away, which I think worsens the behaviour. Whilst most people would address the why, she's more likely to criticise it as a behavioural problem in me.
I know it's not though.

In certain moments it's easy to get lost in that. If you're self aware, you try to look for what you're doing that causes this. Especially when you are so frequently having that reinforced. Even an intelligent person can be vulnerable to this I think. Which I hope I am.

It's exhausting. I feel like I am just getting through life, despite probably having the biggest output I ever have had to. I try to make decisions so positive that it is practically objective. No matter what, it is met with similar behaviours.

If I defend my position, I'm mean. If I speak with any intent, I'm raising my voice. I've even noticed If I defend myself, even with just a slightly mildly impassioned tone, she mentions my height.

I am 6'3. If I say to her "you cannot just say these things and then expect me to be happy when you need me to be", she will say that I am "towering over her shouting". We are taking about zero raised voice. Just talking with intent.

I am so bored of this.

Phew-ThatWasClose
Most of us can relate to being wrong all the time. And the twisted logic. My ex used to tell me I had "wild eyes" and that scared her because as a male I was naturally stronger. Utterly ignoring the fact that I had "wild eyes" because she had been harping on me for half an hour and I'd been asking politely for her to stop for 29 minutes. I

could literally be covering my ears rocking in place chanting "pleasestoppleasestoppleasestoppleasestop" and she would claim I was disrespectful. That's not disrespect, that's a breakdown. :)

After a while the constant negativity just struck me as a game. She didn't even think about what I'd said. She just instantly said "No" and followed with any random reason why I was wrong. It didn't even have to make sense. And If I countered with reason she could always fall back on "I'm not comfortable with that."

My ex also had more acceptance of conflict in front of the kids. She would talk low so the kids wouldn't hear and say the most vile stuff. If I responded in even a normal volume she would say "not in front of the kids." Just an excuse to berate and belittle. It felt like a hostage taking. She set the rules.

Just walk away (p.107). You got it right - it's boring. The PMDD is lazy and it just goes for the jugular every time. The argument is going to play out the same way. Nothing will be resolved. Nothing will be accomplished. It's just the same old same old. The PMDD wants to hurt you and it'll run through greatest hits until it you take the bait. Just walk.

organicHack
Very possibly both PMDD and Borderline (or something else). Needs professional help immediately.

Comradepatrick
I'm also not sure this is PMDD.

My ex was so tired all the time, it became her dominant personality trait. She was constantly struggling to make it through whatever parenting activity we had in front of us, so she could go lie down and have a glass of wine, or smoke cannabis, or whatever. I picked up more and more of the parenting slack, until she asked me for a divorce. Now she gets the break she's been wanting! Half time with our kids, leaves her plenty of time to do her own thing, which I presume is sleep.

Tubular_Jeeves126OP
The odd thing is I don't think she'd divorce me. I think that's the last thing she wants. She seems most reactive when I am fine by myself. That I don't have big demands. I got exhausted by it. I think I talk less,

engage less. Nothing good can come of any of it.

If she divorced me, I'd probably somehow get more free time, more peace, and be healthier. How often is that true of a break up?

I am certain PMDD is there. She has a diagnosis, and I work in pharma, so I can validate to a degree with a reasonably informed opinion. I think it's not the only thing at play though. A lot of these behaviours cross over with her mother. I do notice that her dad doesn't speak or engage much. Possibly finds it wiser not to.

Prior_Thot
PMDD and bipolar are commonly misdiagnosed as one another. I would strongly suggest she get another opinion. As someone with PMDD (but I'm only mean to myself) I have at least one "good week" a month. It sounds like your wife has something else going on, or a co-morbidity.

CompetitiveRub4272
Have you tried couples therapy?

Stars3000
If this goes on during follicular then it definitely sounds like she could have a cluster B personality disorder - borderline personality disorder and probably attachment issues. Who knows maybe bipolar could be mixed in as well like someone said. ideally she should get evaluated by a psychologist and undergo therapy.

I Hate You Don't Leave Me[4] is a good book on understanding borderline personality disorder and your description of this situation resonates with the title of the book.

In my experience (former occupational therapist who worked with adults in various settings and exposure to mental health system due to family etc), people don't exactly fit the description of these disorders and there can be overlap. Definitely sounds more than PMDD and she needs therapy.

Prestigious-Tea6514
It seems like you ard expending a lot of energy arguing and keeping score. I also see some black and shite thinking. Does she just shop, or

---

4   https://a.co/d/7rUY07r

does she parent and teach your lovely son and try to plan events to connect with you? PMDD has nothing to do with this. Please see a marriage counselor.

Tubular_Jeeves126 OP
For someone who used the term "black and shite" thinking, you sure picked a side.

Prestigious-Tea6514
It was a typo but it tracks. You have more grievances than Martin Luther.

Tubular_Jeeves126 OP
It's interesting. I came here for help with something. I have people around me who see how bad it takes a toll. I wanted to understand from people who have seen the toll that PMDD episodes take, and how being non-confrontational does not seem to help. Being quiet becomes the crime. Going somewhere else is hostility by absence
.

I thought perhaps I may be able to be completely honest with people not close to the situation.

One of us here is throwing insults. The other is not.

Phew-ThatWasClose Mod
This is the partner's safe space. There are several women with PMDD who provide a helpful considerate perspective over here. This is not that.

Phew-ThatWasClose Mod – June 23, 2025
This has been living rent free in my head for five days now and I want it out. Have you noticed that the people who whine the most about "keeping score" are the people with the biggest deficits? A lot of us wake up one day and realize we lost ourselves because we *didn't* keep score and there was never anything for us. Where did we go? Why is our cup empty? Why is the score so lopsided?

OP is running as fast as he can and she's just piling on more derision. Then you want to "both sides" it and claim it's nothing to do with PMDD? Read the sub. Same pattern over and over and over. We're meant to be a team. We're meant to be looking out for each other. If one partner is working for the team and the other is looking after themselves … something is missing.

I get that it's a disorder and I get that she's in pain and I get that it *feels* real during the dysphoria. But it's not real and during follicular that needs to be acknowledged and steps need to be taken. So sure, the partnership is only unbalanced half the time. That's **half** the time. Steps need to be taken to correct that and if the dismissive bullshit from luteal is just normalized into follicular the partnership is over.

Saying it's nothing to do with PMDD and marriage counseling is the answer is just delaying the end. In my experience marriage counselors also want to "both sides" it because they want the team to just communicate better. But with PMDD in the mix nothing will change if she doesn't do the work. As it stands now OP is doing all the heavy lifting and marriage counseling that doesn't recognize that will fail. But marriage counseling that does recognize the imbalance will seem biased to her so she'll quit.

They both need individual therapy to address their individual trauma and she needs to actually treat her diagnosed condition.

Wrote this more to help me work through it, but sheesh. OP complains he's being abused and presents the receipts and you want to talk about how complainy he is. Did you miss the abuse part?

> Prestigious-Tea6514
> Can you point me to the part that explains in detail how OP is being abused? If the chief complaint is abuse then there is a lot of extraneous information. A partner being more tired than you are is not abuse. Helping your partner with their CV is not abuse. Being a teacher is not abuse. Saving your son is not abuse.
>
> Subtracting that, what's left is a lot of negativity and possible verbal abuse. I found OP's post belittling toward his wife. Does he really think she gets all her ideas from junk TV? Does she really not allow him to be proud? How can you keep someone from being proud? We also don't know manner, frequency etc. Screaming and yelling is much worse than just being negative.
>
> I think OP should do what most men with unpleasant wives do. Have an affair, preferrably with someone younger. Tell her your problems, get some action and let her stroke your ego for now.
>
> > Phew-ThatWasClose Mod

> Please don't comment over here anymore.

TheChromasphere
It sounds like there's more going on than PMDD and/or that her existing coping mechanisms are straining your relationship and hurting you.

That needs to be addressed and to change. If you think she really does want to stay together, and you do as well, I think counseling / therapy might help you figure out how to shift things to be more sustainable for you. (for both of you— the not wanting you to be happy alone sounds controlling and insecure). If it's more of a situation of her being okay with living at your expense, but she is a good mother, maybe you could coparent well together but would do better separated? Please take care of yourself as best as you can— you're a main example for your kid of how to do that and how to have intimate relationships. Good luck.

Letstalkaboutbpd – July 18, 2025
Honest question, why are you still in this relationship? It sounds truly awful.

At this point does diagnosing her issues really change anything? Many people end toxic relationships and go on to find healthier partners.

I'm not minimizing how hard this might be, but I got depressed just reading your post and imagining your life. You seem like an intelligent successful guy. You don't have to continue trying to find solutions to appease someone who treats you like this.

Also worth mentioning this sounds more like BPD than PMDD to me and I've experienced relationships with women with both disorders. They are very similar with overlapping symptoms but PMDD happens like clockwork every month whereas BPD can happen at literally anytime.

> Tubular_Jeeves126OP
> It's a fair question. I know about BPD, I actually think there is more than one thing going on I agree. I don't think it's BPD though. I think there is some kind of undiagnosed personality disorder at play, but PMDD is definitely in there.
>
> I am in the relationship because of my son. She is good with my son, absolutely adores him. He's incredibly cute, but Down Syndrome can be challenging. In the back of my mind I sometimes question "what happens when he's not as cute anymore".

No matter how present I try to be as a father, I cannot predict her reaction to a separation. The unknown of me not being within the same household/family unit is a unique aspect of my situation that not many could identify with. Right now, I can be a source of positive from him up close. He does not experience any of the PMDD behaviours from her. These things hit me when he's in bed, at nursery, stuff like that.

I have gotten excellent at knowing when to go to the gym, so he is currently unaffected.

The reasoning I have in my head is "if I stay, I suffer the pattern. If I go, maybe he does".

Whilst I've expressed my unhappiness here to a group of people who are at least somewhat removed, at home, I am a very intentionally positive presence. It's tiring but I seem to have near limitless capacity to function through it. I think the hardest part is I can never point myself positively towards a goal. It's all mitigation.

The original post on the sub.[5]

---

5   https://www.reddit.com/r/PMDDpartners/comments/1lca1la

Where do you draw the line for accountability?

Lill1992 - May 28, 2025

This weekend my partner gave me the worst I have ever seen. She threw smartphones on the floor/table to try to break them, she threw a book I had given her which I tried to catch and it hit my wrist and she seemed happy that she had hurt me physically. She was about to throw a small marble statue at me but changed her mind when I flinched and smashed it against a table instead. She was constantly hitting me in my chests with her fingers and it felt like she was trying to get me to be physical with her so she could use it against me. It is my apartment and I took back my keys and helped her drive her stuff to her place after threatening to call the cops, throughout the entire drive she said the most vile things.

She kept sending me messages for the next two days with the most evil things anyone said to me or about me.

I can see in her eyes that it is the PMDD, she really is another being at those times. And after she started to bleed her regrets comes and she wants to get back together.

We had a huge fight over Christmas and I said we either go to therapy or I'm done. We tried one women but she quickly focused on my partner and my partner wanted to change therapist. We changed to another women and she seemed very senior and knowledge, I learned a lot. But over time my partner got tired of it focusing on her and her problems and we stopped.

She does mix the abusers apology with real apologies and when she takes accountability she is very sincere and self-aware, but it really goes in waves. And after this fight I stopped responding and she has taken the initiative to go back to the first therapist and apologized saying a demon had taken hold of her (She means it figurative) but then also said "I attacked you because you did this". She will also try to get medication for PMDD.

So I guess my question are two-fold:
   -What are your strategies for boundaries regarding accountability?

And for the people with PMDD lurking here:
   -What would you say is the best way for me to demand accountability, while still acknowledging that the vileness are being driven by a sickness. I compare it a lot with alcoholics where I would not judge an alcoholic by there actions while influenced, and I don't want to make her feel ashamed for actions outside of her control.

The base fixation she has is thinking that I am in love with one of my closest friends partner. I only meet him 4-5 times a year as he lives 5 hours away and I only meet her roughly half of those times. She thought we interacted with each other on a regular basis so I showed my message history with her and it is around 8 messages over a time of 10 years, all of them being about gifts to my friend. This time she was convinced I have fathered their children all tough the first time I meet her she was pregnant and I never spend time with her alone as I am only there to meet my friend and while visiting I live with another friend. Basically the entire scenario is insane and both therapist has tried to find ways to reach her on this but it goes deep in her.

I apologize for the long text, I have been lurking in these forums for a while and guess I needed to get stuff of my chest.

VacationPractice406
That is awful and I'm so sorry you're going through this. It is good she actually tried therapy and is wanting to try medications, my partner wouldn't even entertain therapy. The throwing things at you and physical abuse is where I would stop. I don't know how you get accountability from them. I'd read here that there can be overlap with borderline and narcissistic personality disorders. For me, borderline made so much sense with my partners behavior and actions. Always shifting blame, never accountable. If I brought up her bad behavior it was justified by her because it was my fault she did that.

Honestly I don't have an answer. My partner broke up with me, she's done this monthly but after the cruel things she said I think she's done. At least you live apart as they would make seperation easier. Your gf really needs treatment to see if that can do anything, as I've read therapy alone may not be a solution.

Take space. Consider your feelings about things. As much as we love them, sometimes it's too much of a strain on ourselves to put up with

dianamxxx
you can't demand accountability from someone who is unwilling to take it and she's left two therapists because she refuses to have the mirror held up. this new therapist will likely be the same and if by some chance she will now listen she needs space to work through her issues and seek medication etc. as wanting change after you've behaved awfully doesn't equate to actual change especially as you can see from her language around what she did.

her behaviour has escalated into physical abuse. for your own safety end this. wish her well but get out.

LizzingWithPMDD
Having PMDD is not her fault — but it is her responsibility.

If she acts or speaks abusively during luteal or not, it's still abuse. You can and should draw boundaries on mental, emotional, and physical abuse — no matter the gender of the abused partner. Your descriptions of her roughly pushing at you (whether to goad you into hitting back or not) is a hard line, PMDD or not. Period.

To be frank on a separated but related note, I think your partner needs to focus on finding the treatments and therapies she needs to better manage her PMDD. This could take some time and is perhaps best done solo. Unless you two have complex ties via marriage, children, or property (house, etc.), I'd recommend moving on and also working with your own therapist to process this relationship so you are happier and healthier for the next.

Virtual_Lunch6331
Leave if you can. It will only get worse.

Phew-ThatWasClose
I stayed far too long because I didn't recognize the verbal abuse for what it was. My ex never got physical and that was my red line. In hindsight I think I was just rationalizing so I wouldn't have to make the hard call. It was after I finally did leave that she got the help she needed.

Alcoholism is a disease, PMDD is a disorder, the comparison is fair to a point. Because we love them we can forgive more than we should. But if a drunk wreaks havoc while under the influence they best seek treatment once sober to get that under control. Same for PMDD. If luteal wreaks havoc and that's outside her control she'd best seek treatment during follicular when it is in her control. Doing nothing about it during follicular, knowing the monster will take over next luteal and hurt the people she loves … that is not okay.

Fundamentally PMDD is chemistry. Therapy can help long term but therapy and will power can only do so much. The gold standard for treatment (p.22) is a Combined Oral Contraceptive taken continuously and a low dose SSRI taken during luteal only (p.26). The second thing they test for when <u>diagnosing</u> (p.18) PMDD is <u>vitamin and mineral deficiencies</u> (p.284) so that "should" already be sorted. If not get that done now.

The particular fixation is irrelevant. If it wasn't that it would be something else. It's a deep insecurity and her therapist can help her dive into where that is coming from. Childhood trauma would be my guess. Point is don't waste your time arguing about it. Even if you "prove" her wrong the PMDD will just shift to something else. Words have power and time spent arguing is time spent reinforcing the lie.

Where you draw the line with untreated unmanaged PMDD is immediately. As soon as you see it in her eyes, as soon as you hear it in her voice, as soon as you feel the vibe in the air, Walk Away. Science has shown the best way to deal with anger is to <u>take a time out</u> (p.107). She'll calm down a lot faster without a target. She may still text the vileness but at least you don't hear it.

AND … if it's escalated to where you have to threaten to call the police to get her out your apartment you are not safe. Now the police are an option. Don't be alone with her during luteal without an exit strategy, and take the exit the instant things get even a little off. Things can get dangerous quickly. Imagine she had thrown that statue. I spent a night in jail because my ex hurt *herself* in my house. Try explaining that to the cops when you're amped up on adrenaline.

Socalwarrior485
You made me do it is an abusers line.

Sundays_Beast
Leave. Now. It's not worth it. How could being single possibly be worse than this?

Specific-Rest1631
There's no such thing as accountability, and there's especially no such thing as demanding it. Forget you ever heard that word. The only thing that exists is boundaries - the boundary between what you are willing to do, and what you are not willing to do. Right now you are willing to have a marble statue thrown at your head. That's because you're being abused, and abusers train your nervous system to be afraid to leave. This woman's physical and mental healing are not your responsibility. It might be very sad for you that you two met at a time in your life where your arc

of healing doesn't line up with hers, but continuing to suffer WILL NOT
HELP HER. I know this seems cruel but take it from someone who
wasted many good years in someone else's healing journey before
realizing that if anything I was holding her back.

LumpyTest1739
Pmdd sufferer here. I'm sorry you are going through that.

That's abuse, and pmdd is no justification for that. One thing is to say
something mean once, another thing is physical violence and days of vile
things. That's not pmdd, it's pmdd exacerbating abuse.

Real accountability comes with action. Is she in treatment? Is she trying
medications, exercise, meditation, supplements, looking for a different
therapist, reading books/listening to podcasts together, working with you
in strategies to deal with the episodes? That's what it means to take
accountability… otherwise it's an empty apology.

BitterActuary3062
Hi. I have PMDD & so did my mother. Growing up I was terrified of her
because she was so horrible to me. But I learned that my mother used
her PMDD to excuse & justify her abuse. Please don't let this happen to
you too. You're worth far more than a punching bag.

The original post on the sub.[6]

---

6   https://www.reddit.com/r/PMDDpartners/comments/1kxb2eg

When she won't let you walk away…

Icy_Resolution5282 - February 2, 2025

This is something I struggle with. I've read the posts on here about walking away and coming back in half an hour once things have cooled down. My PMDD partner will just get into an even bigger rage if I try this and chase me around the house to continue the argument. The other day I walked out of the room after she started screaming and threw a food container at the ground near my feet. She followed me and dragged me by the arm back to where I was to face the music. If I try to leave the house she'll block the way or follow me and leave her keys behind.

We've discussed this outside of lutheal and she agrees in principle that taking space during an argument is healthy but only for a couple of minutes. She feels I'm giving her my back when I walk away, which I presume triggers some sort of abandonedment rage. Also that my movement triggers her (even if I'm just taking a step back).

Ive told her that I'll probably continue walking out if she yells/screams and throws things as it triggers a kind of flight response in me. And she tells me she'll continue chasing me or grabbing me to make me stop moving, because that's apparently the normal thing to do to someone who's anxious and moving erratically?!

Phew-ThatWasClose
One time I was trying to leave there was snow on the ground and I didn't have my shoes which were by the front door. I headed for the door but she blocked me. So I headed for the back door and she blocked me, so I headed for the front door and she blocked me but I got my shoes. Then I headed for the back door and she blocked me but I got it unlocked, then I headed for the front door while putting on one shoe … you get the idea.

Another time she chased me out of the house. I knew from experience she would get in the car if I did so I just started walking. Hands up at a brisk pace. A couple times I had to break into a jog to prevent her from catching up. I had shoes that time, she didn't. She followed for 8 blocks barefoot.

Yes. It gets nutzo sometimes. That is when it is especially important to GTFO. Especially if she's getting physical and you're also getting activated. Things can go south really fast and jail is a very real possibility. Guess how I know. You. Are. Not. Safe. This is the reason it's called a safety plan (p.59).

If she's triggered by you showing your back then back away, hands up, universal peace. You probably want to keep her in line of sight anyway. If she follows you to the other room leave the house. If she follows you out of the house walk around the block. If she's screaming all through the neighborhood that's not on you. If she leaves her keys behind, put a hide a key somewhere. If she has abandonment issues - gee, I wonder why?

You have to take care of you. Put on your own oxygen mask before assisting others. Don't set yourself on fire to keep her warm. Boundaries (p.127) that are not enforced are just suggestions.

If you come back in half an hour, maybe an hour, and she wants to start up again, leave again. It's going to be hard at first. Really hard. And maybe you have to spend that first night on a buddies couch or a motel. Maybe it's "too much drama". Well, good. Bring everything out in the open and talk about it in follicular. The current situation is not sustainable. Something has to change.

Happy to chat if you wish.

Smart_Prior_6534
Your dedication to helping others is admirable. Always here with solid advice.

Icy_Resolution5282 OP
Thank you for all this advice. We have discussed these things during follicular but haven't gotten to the stage of formalising a safety plan. That has to be the next step because it is not sustainable... Recent months have been getting worse.

LonelySound1228
The key is not to just leave during the argument the key is to leave and not return at all.

AcadiaPrimary614
I set my garage up as a safe room and would lock myself in there until she calmed down, before that she would follow me around the house baiting and abusing me until I snapped, then I was the bad guy.

She's medicated now and exercises regularly so these behaviors have stopped.

> THREEFIFTYSE7EN
> What medication is she on? My missus has PMDD and it's slowly destroying our relationship. I'm sick of losing my girl for half the month to this bullshit. Every time it happens, I fall less and less in love with her.

>> jazzysmaxashmone
>> I am on prozac. It has changed my life. Not guarantees that it will work for her, and there can be a period of rough side effects. But my psychiatrist said, "it is the treatment for PMDD" and I am so friggn glad I trusted her and tried it.
>> I hope your gf can find peace. I felt like a monster for so long, but now I realize it's pmdd. I can build from here. I have hope now

>> Instantaneous242
>> My wife (44F) is on norethindrone birth control. Has worked wonders to reduce (Not eliminate) the PMDD tendencies. Wish we had found these meds 15 years ago. I feel like half my marriage was a loss (2 weeks of every month).

Strange-King8917
Yeah man I know exactly what u mean. Ine did that to me it was horrible, trying to find a resolution with here for the at three years and this would happen and she'd just run away from trying to find solutions. Anyway enough was enough we are separating for good!!!

Married 11yrs 15yrs together with two young kids. Could not go on anymore. Id rather love in horseshit the rest of my life than cop the emotional and physical abuse that I have for many years. Horrible and to all the guys that stayed in the marriage I so applaud you you are the real heroes like for real. Supermen. Best

beenbagbeagle
It's funny because I'm the one with PMDD but my partner (as supportive as he can be) is the one who leans towards this. I'll recognize when it's getting heated and request space and when he doesn't "allow" it, it's for such and such reason. He's anxious attached and I'm more avoidant

though, so it's like we're both playing to our trigger responses oppositely.

I did think you made this post suggesting that she wouldn't let you leave leave like leave the relationship. And I clicked in thinking "I can totally relate". Every time I suggest separation due to the toxicity and my illness he always demands or begs me to stay. Is this how it is for you too?

Icy_Resolution5282 OP
Thanks, this does sound like opposite trigger responses. She's anxious attached and I'm probably more avoidant. I'd find it much easier to deal with if she'd just send me to the garage.

Sometimes she suggests separation and tells me she hates me and I make her worse etc but I think it's a test. I once left for a night after things got too wild and she was begging me to come back.

Temporary-Swan-4793
I'm (pwPMDD) someone who finds it hard to let my partner leave in a dysregulated way. My partner (also pwPMDD) finds it challenging to communicate that they need space in a healthy way.

We trigger each other's attachment systems and it has led to immense blow out fights.

We are both working on our responses - me to be proactive about taking space when I feel dysregulated (a novel concept) and my partner to identify when they're becoming dysregulated and ask for space in a way that works WITH me and not against me.

It's been very unsuccessful so far but we're continuing to try new strategies to achieve this.

Phew-ThatWasClose
My therapist explained it to me like this (p.114). There's a worksheet and everything. Basically you think about your triggers and preferred responses and write it all down and then say it out loud once a day for thirty days. That's supposed to retrain your brain to be more aware when it happens. Honestly it kinda works. :)

Electrical_Hyena5164

Scientifically, you can't have the conversation in fight flight freeze. So walking away til that's over is the only thing to do. If she has abandonment issues that are triggered by this, she needs to work on those. You can't fix that for her and you can't just cop abuse to spare her abandonment feelings. Ideally, you would say something calm like "I love you but I have to have some space and I will be back.". But I never manage that because I have PTSD. But even though she tries to stop me, it is always better when I actually manage to make myself leave the house.

Secure-Number2732
This is obviously toxic behaviour by her. If she treats you like this just during the pmdd time of her cycle than if you love her stay with her. communicate to her that you are struggling with her symptoms and want to discuss and come up with a plan to manage her pmdd together (when her symptoms have passed.) Try work together to find her root cause. For my partner it's her dysregulated nervous system and she is working on regulating that with a natropath. So I know she is working on it and our relationship won't be like this forever making it easier for me to cope with her pmdd. If she doesn't want to fix her pmdd and she doesn't accept help than leaving her might be the right thing. She should be wanting to help herself for the both of you and people who don't want to help themselves in general are red flags.

LumpyTest1739
Something that could help is setting a clear boundary and expectations. During follicular, have a conversation where you explain how this makes you feel and what you need: ie, you need to take a break and postpone the conversation when things get heated. She needs to agree, because this is a reasonable request.

Now, the implementation is very critical. It's very different if you say: A) I can't take it anymore, I'm leaving, I need a break. B) this conversation is getting too intense and I will not tolerate yelling/name calling/throwing things. I will go for a walk/take a break and I will be back in 2h, and we can talk more then. I love you and we're ok, but I am feeling exhausted and overwhelmed, and not capable of continuing the conversation right now.

Instantaneous242
I'm glad I stumbled upon this thread. I thought I was the only husband whose PMDDing wife didn't let him walk away for a while during an

intense emotional explosion.

The worst is when someone or something will trigger her while we are in the car on the way to somewhere. She just won't stop with the nastiest, vilest things you've ever heard. I can't get away and she won't stop talking. If I stay quiet, it is an issue and if I talk it is an issue. Classic rock and hard place situation.

I don't know how I managed not to crash the car into an overpass.

The original post on the sub.[7]

---

7   https://www.reddit.com/r/PMDDpartners/comments/1igfcle

Appendix

Miscellany that needed to be included but didn't belong anywhere else. :<(

Save your energy, use it for something that makes a difference, like making dinner.

Turns out it's calming things that calm you down.

Science has shown the best way to deal with anger, anybody's anger, is to take a time out.

The couples that make it are the ones that can work together against the common enemy.

DSM-5 Diagnostic Criteria for PMDD

Timing of symptoms

A) In the majority of menstrual cycles, at least 5 symptoms must be present in the final week before the onset of menses, start to improve within a few days after the onset of menses, and become minimal or absent in the week post menses

Symptoms

B) One or more of the following symptoms must be present:

1) Marked affective lability (e.g., mood swings, feeling suddenly sad or tearful, or increased sensitivity to rejection)
2) Marked irritability or anger or increased interpersonal conflicts
3) Markedly depressed mood, feelings of hopelessness, or self-deprecating thoughts
4) Marked anxiety, tension, and/or feelings of being keyed up or on edge

C) One (or more) of the following symptoms must additionally be present to reach a total of 5 symptoms when combined with symptoms from criterion B above

5) Decreased interest in usual activities
6) Subjective difficulty in concentration
7) Lethargy, easy fatigability, or marked lack of energy
8) Marked change in appetite; overeating or specific food cravings
9) Hypersomnia or insomnia
10) A sense of being overwhelmed or out of control
11) Physical symptoms such as breast tenderness or swelling; joint or muscle pain, a sensation of "bloating" or weight gain

Severity

D) The symptoms are associated with clinically significant distress or interference with work, school, usual social activities, or relationships with others.

Consider Other Psychiatric Disorders

E) The disturbance is not merely an exacerbation of the symptoms of another disorder, such as major depressive disorder, panic disorder, persistent depressive disorder (dysthymia) or a personality disorder (although it may co-occur with any of these disorders).

Confirmation of the disorder

F) Criterion A should be confirmed by prospective daily ratings during at least 2 symptomatic cycles (although a provisional diagnosis may be made prior to this confirmation)

Exclude other Medical Explanations

G) The symptoms are not attributable to the physiological effects of a substance (e.g., drug abuse, medication or other treatment) or another medical condition (e.g., hyperthyroidism).

Adapted from: Premenstrual Dysphoric Disorder (Formerly Premenstrual Syndrome)[1] Some formatting (spaces, line returns) added for clarity. Bolding and unnecessary capitalization is original.

Another version at PsychDB[2]
Another version at Wikipedia[3]

---

1   http://www.ncbi.nlm.nih.gov/books/NBK279045
2   http://www.psychdb.com/mood/pmdd#dsm-5-diagnostic-criteria
3   http://en.wikipedia.org/wiki/Premenstrual_dysphoric_disorder#DSM-5

ICD-11 Diagnostic Criteria for PMDD
(Code: GA34.41)

World Health Organization
International Classification of Diseases 11th Revision (January, 2022)

Description

During a majority of menstrual cycles within the past year, a pattern of mood symptoms (depressed mood, irritability), somatic symptoms (lethargy, joint pain, overeating), or cognitive symptoms (concentration difficulties, forgetfulness) that begin several days before the onset of menses, start to improve within a few days after the onset of menses, and then become minimal or absent within approximately 1 week following the onset of menses. The temporal relationship of the symptoms and luteal and menstrual phases of the cycle should ideally be confirmed by a prospective symptom diary over at least two symptomatic menstrual cycles. The symptoms are severe enough to cause significant distress or significant impairment in personal, family, social, educational, occupational or other important areas of functioning and do not represent the exacerbation of a mental disorder.

Essential (Required) Features:

- During a majority of menstrual cycles within the past year, a pattern of mood, somatic, or cognitive symptoms is present that begins several days before the onset of menses, starts to improve within a few days after the onset of menses, and then becomes minimal or absent within approximately 1 week following the onset of menses. The temporal relationship of the symptoms and luteal and menstrual phases of the cycle should ideally be confirmed by a prospective symptom diary over at least two symptomatic menstrual cycles.
- The symptoms include:
  - ► At least one affective symptom such as mood lability, irritability, depressed mood, or anxiety, and
  - ► Additional somatic or cognitive symptom(s) such as lethargy, joint pain, overeating, hypersomnia, breast tenderness, swelling of extremities, concentration difficulties, or forgetfulness.
- The symptoms are not better accounted for by another mental disorder (e.g., a Mood Disorder, an Anxiety or Fear-Related Disorder).
- The symptoms are not a manifestation of another medical condition (e.g., endometriosis, polycystic ovary disease, adrenal system disorders and hyperprolactinemia) and are not due to the

effects of a substance or medication on the central nervous system (e.g., hormone treatment, alcohol), including withdrawal effects (e.g., from stimulants).
- The symptoms result in significant distress or significant impairment in personal, family, social, educational, occupational or other important areas of functioning.

Boundary with Normality (Threshold):
- Mild mood changes (e.g., increased emotional lability, irritability, subjective tension) that occur during late luteal or menstrual phase of the cycle for many women should not be labelled as Premenstrual Dysphoric Disorder. In contrast to Premenstrual Dysphoric Disorder, these symptoms are less intense and do not typically result in significant distress or impairment.

Boundaries with Other Disorders and Conditions (Differential Diagnosis):
- **Boundary with Premenstrual Tension Syndrome:** Many women may experience cyclic emotional, physical, or behavioural symptoms that interfere with their lifestyles during the luteal phase of the menstrual cycle that are appropriately diagnosed and treated as Premenstrual Tension Syndrome. This is in contrast to Premenstrual Dysphoric Disorder, in which the symptoms are considerably more severe and cause significant distress or significant impairment in personal, family, social, educational, occupational or other important areas of functioning.

- **Boundary with other Mental, Behavioural or Neurodevelopmental Disorders including Mood Disorders that are exacerbated premenstrually:** Mood symptoms characteristic of Premenstrual Dysphoric Disorder including depressed mood, irritability, and anxiety can be present in other Mental, Behavioural or Neurodevelopmental Disorders (e.g., Depressive Disorders, Bipolar Disorders, Generalized Anxiety Disorder). Although symptoms of these disorders may be exacerbated during the late luteal and menstrual phases, Premenstrual Dysphoric Disorder is differentiated by the absence of symptoms 1 week post-menses. Because of the difficulty in accurate recall of the relationship between menstrual cycle and the course of symptoms, prospective mood ratings for two consecutive cycles should be considered.

- **Boundary with Dysmenorrhea:** Dysmenorrhea is characterized by cyclic pelvic pain or lower, umbilical, or suprapubic abdominal pain preceding or accompanying menstruation that interferes with daily activities. Unlike Premenstrual Dysphoric Disorder, the onset of Dysmenorrhea is coincident with the start of rather than prior to menses. Furthermore, mood symptoms are not typically associated with this condition.

- **Boundary with the effects of hormones and their synthetic substitutes and antagonists:** Use of hormone treatments, including for contraceptive purposes, may result in unwanted side effects that include mood, somatic, and cognitive symptoms. If symptoms do not persist after cessation of these medications beyond the period when their physiological effects should have subsided a diagnosis of Premenstrual Dysphoric Disorder should not be assigned.

Adapted from ICD-11 for Mortality and Morbidity Statistics[4]

---

4   https://icd.who.int/browse/2024-01/mms/en#1526774088

Should I stay for the kids?

(What are ACEs?)(Take 2)

TasteGlittering4459 – Feb 2, 2025

From the Minnesota Department of Health webpage on ACEs[5]

TL;DR Available at the bottom, denoted by this ❗ emoji

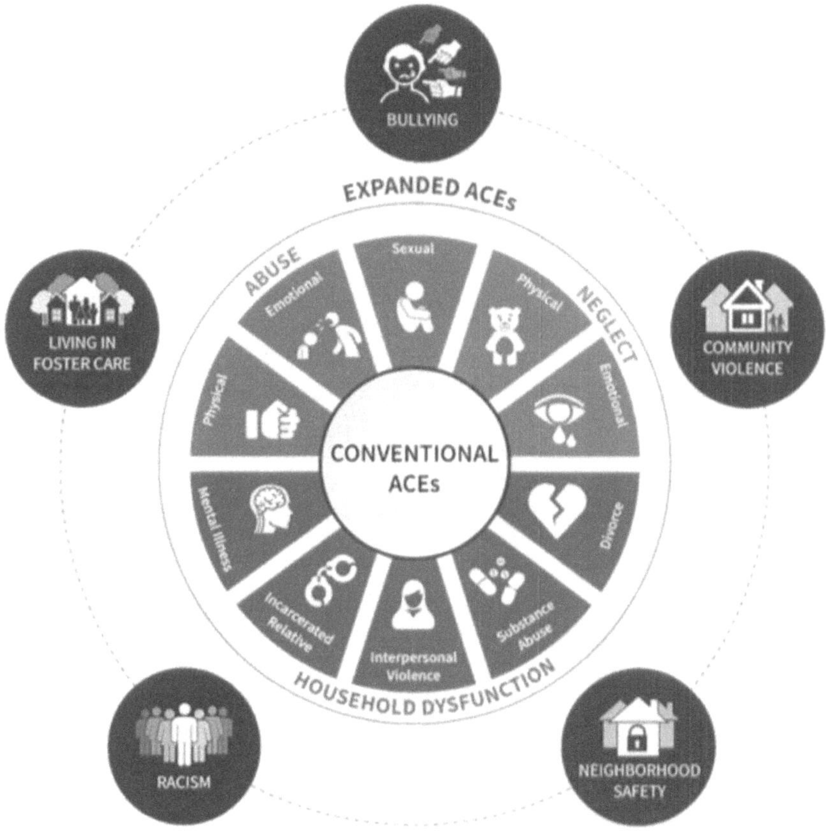

Foreword (feel free to skip) : In the midst of researching for this post, my job was made needlessly harder by the Trump administration's strategy for

5   https://www.health.state.mn.us/communities/ace/index.html

implementing their new guidelines for government websites. For my readers in the US, regardless of how you feel about the current administration, I feel it should be concerning to everyone that information as benign as "people with rough childhoods are more likely to struggle in adulthood and there has been extensive, credible research over the last 30 years to back this assertion up" has been deemed as violating their guidelines. We should all be asking ourselves, *why* was it necessary to immediately dismantle access to this information, and *who* benefits when information like this isn't easily accessible public knowledge. I hate to be political, but in this case I was figuratively slapped in the face with it, *and* I needed to provide context as to why I'm using web archive links. Anyways, onto the post.

So you have kids with your Abusive PMDD partner and have decided to stay for related reasons.

*(Disclaimer: **ABUSIVE** is the important operative word here. If you have kids with your PMDD partner and they aren't abusive, while you may still find this post informative, you are not the primary intended audience. If you're unsure whether your relationship is abusive or not, I encourage you to check out my last post (p.211). It has some infographics about behaviors that are often characteristic of abusive relationships, and other useful information regarding domestic violence. Additionally, I am intentionally assigning no moral judgement to anyone's decision to stay or leave their abusive partner and am kindly requesting that people who comment do the same. It is an incredibly difficult and complicated decision to make when there are children involved, and while well intended, comments encouraging someone to leave their abusive partner can contribute to feelings of toxic shame if not worded carefully. I also want to avoid unintentionally invalidating other's experiences. Only you have access to all the information regarding your situation, and only you can decide whether you believe separation is the right choice for your family.)*

Whether you have decided to stay for the benefits of a 2 parent household, your fears over custody, or anything else, this post is for you. A common misconception in our culture (that I have also seen perpetuated at times in this subreddit) is that the benefits to children of a 2 parent household outweigh the benefits of leaving, except for in the most 'extreme' abuse situations. To counter this, I would like to present some information that isn't necessarily common knowledge: a relatively new-ish psychological concept called **ACEs**. The research on ACEs shows that the pervasive idea of 2 parent households being the *only* and/or *best* way for children to have positive life outcomes lacks critically important nuance. My intention in sharing this information is not to, in any way, imply people who decide to stay with their partner for their child's wellbeing are in the wrong. Instead, it is to share information that I believe (if one was previously unaware of it) may strongly influence the call they decide to make.

What are ACEs?

<u>Quick Facts</u>[6]

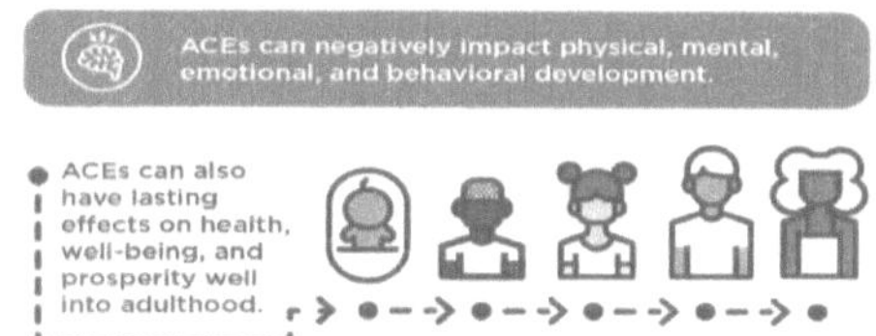

ACE stands for *Adverse Childhood Experience.* They are defined as traumatic events that can impact a child's development that occur between the ages of 0 and 17.

The original ACE studies were conducted by <u>CDC-Kaiser Permanente</u>[7] from 1995-1997. After researchers identified negative experiences children may go through that they believed could influence life outcomes, and defining them as ACEs, Kaiser Permanente conducted surveys based on those factors across 17,000+ participants over 2 years. Their research found that ACEs are common across all populations, and nearly two-thirds of their participants had experienced at least one ACE, among other findings. The discovery from this study that is the most relevant to this post is the correlation between the number of ACEs experienced by children and the risk of negative outcomes in adulthood. There have been many studies following the CDC-Kaiser Permanente study that support and expand upon their findings, with some ACE studies continuing to the present day.

6   https://drive.google.com/file/d/10o8gckC0Tzqfz-r-75gK5FM-TWq0rZJE/view?usp=sharing
7   https://web.archive.org/web/20241216104023/https://www.cdc.gov/violenceprevention/
     aces/about.html

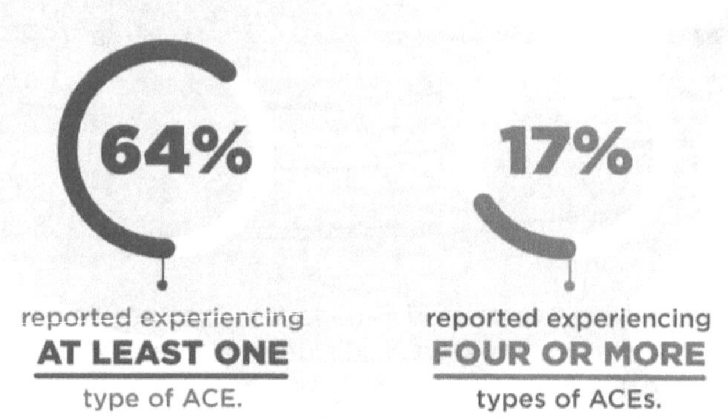

The Minnesota Department of Health has a good, succinct list[8] of experiences that are considered ACEs on their website. While the federal CDC websites about ACEs also have (or, had) similar lists, I think the list provided by The Minnesota Department of Health is the best one to reference. It is specific enough to not leave too much up to interpretation, but open enough to easily extrapolate different ways these factors may present in one's life. I also ripped the infographic at the top of this post from their website. This is their list:

- Abuse (Physical, Emotional, or Sexual)
- Neglect (Physical Or Emotional)
- Household Challenges (Financial Hardship, Drug Addiction, Etc)
- Living with a parent or caregiver with severe mental health challenges
- Discrimination
- Feeling unsafe in their neighborhood
- Bullying
- Witnessing Violence

Why does it matter?

The findings from studies about ACEs consistently show that, the more ACEs a child has, the higher their risk is of experiencing negative/adverse outcomes in adulthood . Per the CDC:

---

8   https://www.health.state.mn.us/communities/ace/basics.html

"ACEs can have lasting effects on health and well-being in childhood and life opportunities well into adulthood. Life opportunities include things like education and job potential. These experiences can increase the risks of injury, sexually transmitted infections, and involvement in sex trafficking. They can also increase risks for maternal and child health problems including teen pregnancy, pregnancy complications, and fetal death. Also included are a range of chronic diseases and leading causes of death, such as cancer, diabetes, heart disease, and suicide"

A few years after the initial ACE studies were completed, Harvard

ACEs Can Increase Risk for Disease, Early Death, and Poor Social Outcomes

Research shows that **experiencing a higher number of ACEs is** associated with **many of the leading causes of death** like heart disease and cancer.

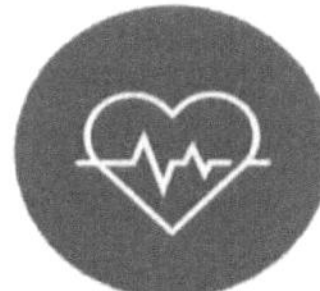

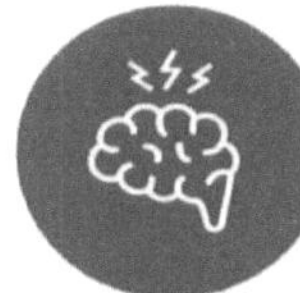

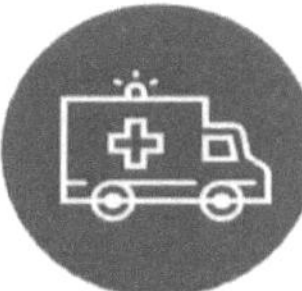

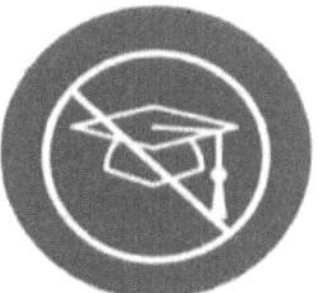

CHRONIC HEALTH CONDITIONS	MENTAL HEALTH CONDITIONS AND SUBSTANCE USE DISORDERS	HEALTH RISK BEHAVIORS	SOCIAL OUTCOMES
• Coronary heart disease • Stroke • Asthma • Chronic obstructive pulmonary disease (COPD) • Cancer • Kidney disease • Diabetes • Obesity	• Depression • Substance use disorder including alcohol, opioids, and tobacco	• Smoking • Excessive alcohol use • Substance misuse • Physical inactivity • Risky sexual behavior • Suicidal thoughts and behavior	• Lack of health insurance • Unemployment • Less than high school diploma or equivalent education

University's National Scientific Council on the Developing Child created the term *Toxic Stress* to "describe extensive, scientific knowledge about the effects of excessive activation of stress response systems on a child's developing brain, as well as the immune system, metabolic regulatory systems, and cardiovascular system." They also found that "experiencing ACEs triggers all of these interacting stress response systems."

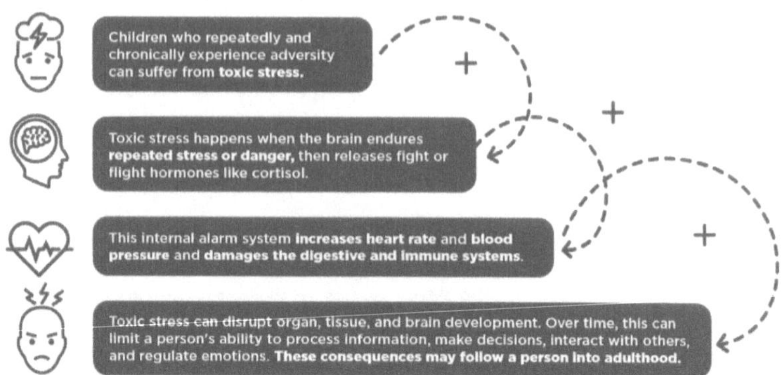

It's important to remember that stress itself is not an inherently bad thing. Expecting to make one's way through life without experiencing a single stressor would be considered delusional, as we all know stress is a natural part of the ebb and flow of life. Additionally, successfully navigating through stressful situations can help develop problem solving skills and foster resilience. I don't think any well adjusted person would advocate for trying to keep a kid sheltered in a protective bubble. It's the scale of the stress, and the resulting cumulative effects of stress at that scale, that makes ACEs so detrimental. Without protective factors in place to help counter the negative effect of ACEs, these cumulative effects can easily develop into an overactive stress response, which is incredibly hard on the developing body and mind. The CDC lists some potential outcomes from toxic stress:

"Children growing up with toxic stress may have difficulty forming healthy and stable relationships. They may also have unstable work histories as adults and struggle with finances, jobs, and depression throughout life. These effects can also be passed on to their own children[...]"

ACEs Can Echo Across Generations

The consequences of ACEs can **be passed down from one generation to the next** if children don't have protective buffers like...

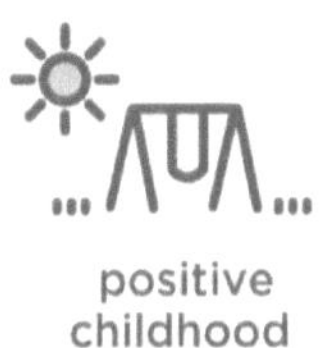

positive childhood experiences

OR

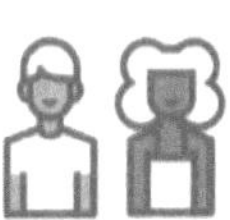

a caring adult in their lives.

Also, when families experience **historical and systemic racism** or living in **poverty for generations**, the effects of ACEs **can add up over time.**

What are protective factors?

Simply put, protective factors are things in a child's life that can help mitigate the effects of ACEs. You may still decide, even after you finish reading this post, that leaving would be more detrimental to your child than staying. After all, Divorce is considered an ACE too. Regardless of what you decide, there are protective factors you can put into place to help your child cope with their home situation. To better understand protective factors, I think it is important to also know some risk factors that the CDC associates with an increased likelihood of experiencing and ACE:

Individual and Family Risk Factors:
- Families experiencing caregiving challenges due to a child with special needs
- Children and youth who don't feel close to their parents and feel like they can't talk to them about their feelings
- Youth who start dating/engaging in sexual activity early
- Children with no or few friends, or friends that engage in delinquent behavior
- Families with caregivers who have a limited understanding of children's needs or development
- Families or caregivers that were abused or neglected as children
- Families with young caregivers or single parents
- Families with low income
- Families with adults with low levels of education
- Families experiencing high levels of parenting stress or economic stress
- Families with caregivers who use spanking or other forms of corporal punishment for discipline
- Families with inconsistent discipline and/or low levels of parental monitoring and supervision

- Families that are isolated and not connected to other people (extended family, friends, neighbors)
- Families with high conflict and negative communication styles.

Community Risk Factors:
- Communities with high rates of violence and crime
- Communities with high rates of poverty and limited educational and economic opportunities
- Communities with high unemployment rates
- Communities with easy access to drugs and alcohol
- Communities where neighbors don't know and look out for each other and there is low community involvement among residents
- Communities with few community activities for young people
- Communities with unstable housing and where residents move frequently
- Communities where families frequently experience food insecurity
- Communities with high levels of social and environmental disorder

I'm sure just through reading these, you can think of a few strategies to help mitigate them. A lot of it is common sense stuff like trying to reside in a safe community and being involved in your child's life. The CDC also provides a list of protective factors:

Individual and Family Protective Factors:
- Families who create safe, stable and nurturing relationships meaning children have a consistent family life where they are safe, taken care of, and supported
- Children who have positive friendships and peer networks
- Children who do well in school
- Children who have caring adults outside the family who act as mentors and role models
- Families where caregivers can meet basic needs of food, shelter, and health services for children
- Families where caregivers have college degrees or higher
- Families where caregivers have steady employment
- Families with strong social support networks and positive relationships with the people around them
- Families where caregivers engage in parental monitoring, supervision, and enforcement of rules
- Families where caregivers/adults work through conflict peacefully
- Families where caregivers help children work through problems
- Families that engage in fun positive activities together
- Families that encourage the importance of school for children

Community protective factors:
- Communities where families have access to economic and financial

help

- Communities where families have access to health care and mental health services
- Communities with access to safe, stable housing
- Communities where families have access to safe and nurturing childcare
- Communities where families have access to safe, engaging after school programs and activities
- Communities where families have access to a high quality pre-school
- Communities where adults have work opportunities with family friendly policies.
- Communities with strong partnership between the community and business, health care, government, and other sectors
- Communities where residents feel connected to each other and are involved in the community
- Communities where violence is not acceptable or tolerated

We Can Create Positive Childhood Experiences

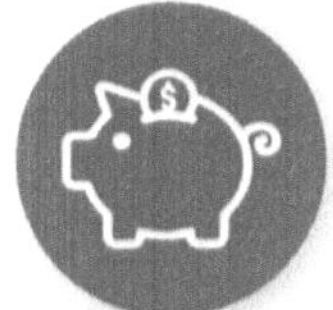

Strengthen families' financial stability

- Paid time off
- Child tax credits
- Flexible and consistent work schedules

Promote social norms that protect against violence

- Positive parenting practices
- Prevention efforts involving men and boys

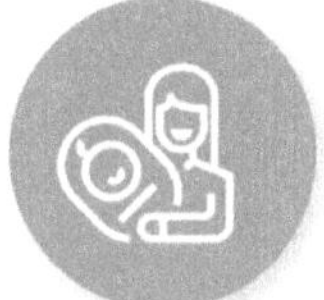

Help kids have a good start

- Early learning programs
- Affordable preschool and childcare programs

Teach healthy relationship skills

- Conflict resolution
- Negative feeling management
- Pressure from peers
- Healthy non-violent dating relationships

Connect youth with activities and caring adults

- School or community mentoring programs
- After-school activities

Intervene to lessen immediate and long-term harms

- ACEs education
- Therapy
- Family-centered treatment for substance abuse

Some of these are more within our control and/or more actionable than others. Regardless of that or the situation you're in, there are still supports that you can put in place for your child. The research shows these supports will help them thrive in spite of adversity. The National Scientific Council on the Developing Child emphasizes the importance of "supportive relationships with adults to provide buffering protection" - meaning, just being there and actively trying to be a good parent for your kid helps them out a lot. Making an active effort to be involved in your surrounding community is another powerful protective factor, as it would have a two-fold effect of actively helping your child in the present and helping ensure they have a positive future.

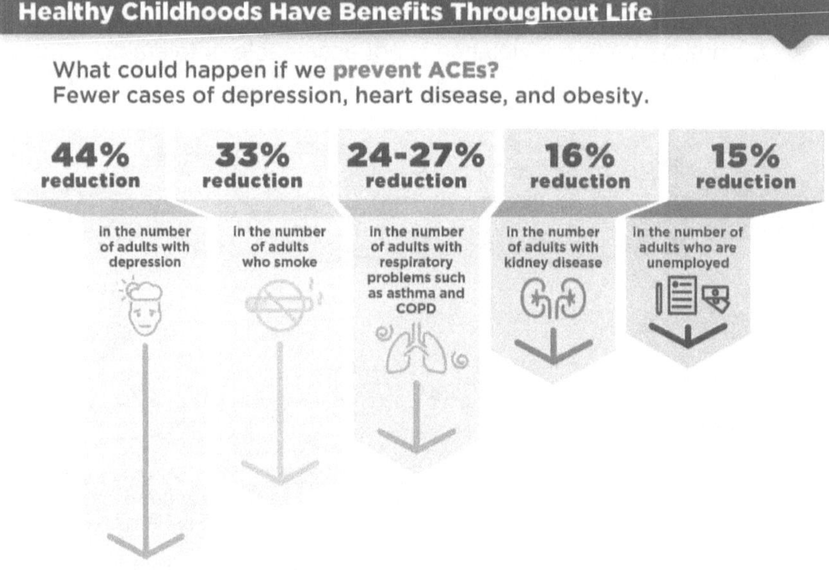

And that's the end of my primer on ACEs as it applies to partners of those with PMDD. I hope it was helpful and informative. If you're interested in community involvement around ACEs, I reuploaded some of the resources that were previously available through the CDC websites onto my google[9] drive. Additionally, I reuploaded this very helpful pdf[10] that I recommend to those who want more info or an easily shareable format.

---

9   https://drive.google.com/drive/folders/1jtlzQrEHYdvz94yQzWKGHkneCCktDF-F?usp=drive_link

10 https://drive.google.com/file/d/1ryZwrpDMZAG8cKRfE7O8ojgWij0h50X1/view?usp=sharing

! ! ! ! ! TL;DR - Experiencing trauma as a child makes you more likely to have negative outcomes in adulthood, and staying with your abusive partner just to make sure your kid has a 2 parent household may be a misguided decision. When deciding what you want to do, consider the impact of prolonged stress on your child's development, and ways you could mitigate that stress. ! ! ! ! !

Sources:

- ACE Wheel Infographic[11]
- All other Infographics[12]
- CDC-Kaiser Study Info[13]
- National Scientific Council on the Developing Child Info[14]
- CDC's About ACEs Website[15]
- CDC's VitalSigns about ACEs[16]
- VetoViolence (CDC site)[17]
- Minnesota Department of Health ACE webpage[18]

---

11 https://www.health.state.mn.us/communities/ace/basics.html
12 https://web.archive.org/web/20240929112200mp_/https://www.cdc.gov/aces/communication-resources/index.html
13 https://web.archive.org/web/20241216104023/https://www.cdc.gov/violenceprevention/aces/about.html
14 https://developingchild.harvard.edu/resources/infographics/aces-and-toxic-stress-frequently-asked-questions/
15 https://web.archive.org/web/20241231044035/https://www.cdc.gov/aces/about/index.html
16 https://web.archive.org/web/20240923173432/https://www.cdc.gov/vitalsigns/aces/index.html
17 https://web.archive.org/web/20240927071828/https://vetoviolence.cdc.gov/apps/aces-infographic/
18 https://www.health.state.mn.us/communities/ace/basics.html

Vitamins and Supplements

Have your partner get tested for vitamin and mineral deficiencies. This is important![19] For whatever reason Doctors don't tend to do this. Sometimes people who have been suffering for years report they got tested, started taking a supplement, and their symptoms went away. My ex was one of those people. Do this first!

Iron is especially important and all people who menstruate lose a substantial amount of iron every month. For some reason ferritin levels are considered "normal" if they are above 15 ug/L, but symptoms of Iron Deficiency Without Anemia[20] (IDWA) can occur even with levels in the 80s. Ferritin levels are not considered dangerous until they are in the 200's and IDWA symptoms are treated[21] by targeting a level of 100 ug/L. So when you get tested *pay attention to your ferritin level* and ask your doctor about it.

Some in the medical community are starting to come around. As of fall 2024 Ontario has changed their guidelines[22] to designate ferritin levels below 20 ug/l as iron deficiency, 20-50 ug/L as probable iron deficiency and 50-100 ug/L as possible iron deficiency. They (Ontario) have a whole dedicated website which includes the catchy slogan "Just because iron deficiency is common doesn't mean it's normal" and lists *being female* as a risk factor for iron deficiency.

Follow label directions and ask a doctor about anything that might interfere with medications your partner is already taking. Usually prescriptions come with a sheet that lists things to avoid. E.g.: people who take thyroid medicine can't eat grapefruit. :)

Calcium is the only officially recommended supplement for PMDD in the new guidelines from The American College of Obstetricians and Gynocologists. All women need calcium to guard against Osteoporosis. Women with PMDD need more.[23] Moreover a Combined Oral Contraceptive is a first tier treatment for PMDD and birth control leaches calcium from the body. Don't overdo, but make sure you get enough.

The Royal College of Obstetricians and Gynaecologists recommends primrose oil, vitamin B6, and magnesium.

B6, B12, Iron[24], Magnesium, Vitamin D and sometimes Zinc and sometimes

---

19 http://www.reddit.com/r/PMDD/comments/1f6vlst
20 http://www.reddit.com/r/PMDD/comments/1g13ask
21 http://pmc.ncbi.nlm.nih.gov/articles/PMC8002799
22 http://www.lifelabs.com/notification/update-to-reporting-of-ferritin-in-ontario
23 http://www.reddit.com/r/PMDD/comments/s2n6b9
24 http://www.reddit.com/r/PMDD/comments/1fi4a8w

Potasium[25] seem to top everyone's list. A good start in the "can't hurt might help" category while you wait for your appointment/tests. And Vitamin C is good for everything so throw that in.

Read this thread about Magnesium[26]
And this one as well.[27]
Read this thread about Vitamin D[28]
Here's an entire thread about sleep[29]
And another one[30]
Here's an entire thread about staying hydrated[31]
Here's an entire thread about exercise[32]

The standard of care (p.22) is Birth Control and an SSRI. The least medicated option is *just* a low dose intermittent SSRI (p.26). Folks who can't for some reason, or would like to try something gentler first, turn to supplements. There are often reports in the PMDD sub of somebody who "tried everything else" and suddenly found the one that clicked.

Even with supplements[33] follow label directions. Everybody is different and if something doesn't work for you try something else. Don't double the dose thinking that'll help. Maybe it's "just a supplement" but too much can still be dangerous. A friend of mine points out that modern medicines started out as supplements so take appropriate care.

A note on Pepcid AC: There is no evidence[34] Pepcid AC helps with PMDD. There is, however, evidence it helps with other things (like MCAS) that have similar symptoms. It is helpful to enough people who believe they have PMDD that it has caused quite some controversy. The antihistamine true believers have even started their own sub at r/PMDDSharing.[35] Since it's cheap, off the shelf, and probably already in your medicine cabinet, give it a try. If it helps get tested for MCAS.

Below is a random list brazenly lifted from people's success stories on the PMDD sub. The PMDD wiki has a similar list[36] that is more scientific.

---

25 http://iapmd.org/blog-posts/2017/10/16/pmdd-and-potassium
26 http://www.reddit.com/r/PMDD/comments/1cfxetw
27 http://www.reddit.com/r/PMDD/comments/1e8psse
28 http://www.reddit.com/r/PMDD/comments/1d8wsvs
29 http://www.reddit.com/r/PMDD/comments/1dw4cqw
30 http://www.reddit.com/r/PMDD/comments/1hstqs7
31 http://www.reddit.com/r/PMDD/comments/1fypbz2
32 http://www.reddit.com/r/PMDD/comments/1g2o4k9
33 http://www.reddit.com/r/PMDD/comments/1enfr50
34 https://www.reddit.com/r/PMDD/comments/1h28plt
35 https://www.reddit.com/r/PMDDSharing/
36 https://www.reddit.com/r/PMDD/wiki/index/vitamins_supplements/

The Last Desperate Flail

Additionally some people have contributed <u>more detailed accounts</u>[37] of what works for them.

Nutrition Movement Medicine Mindfulness There are many strategies we must apply…often all of them need to be done for relief. Thinking happy thoughts wont work, with all due respect.

I bought a red bracelet to wear in my window. This means my period protocol is on. I forget when I am in my window and my thoughts feel so real. My bracelet will remind me that my feelings don't align with the facts.

I manage a small team of 4 and we have a crocheted "positive pickle" in our office. The idea is that if you're having a rough one, keep <u>positive pickle</u>[38] at your desk so the rest of the team know to be extra gentle

---

Quitting caffeine improved my symptoms significantly.
No caffeine, 50mg sertraline (Zoloft) every day. I no longer have pmdd symptoms
The days I drink tea instead of coffee — I feel 70% better and more optimistic.
Tea contains theanine. Earl Grey also has bergamot.
BUT LITERALLY JUST TRY <u>GREEN TEA</u>[39] INSTEAD OF COFFEE FOR A FEW DAYS. its like my brain just calmed tf down!!!
Spearmint tea. Drinking this a few times a week has completely stopped my cystic acne.
It's been three months since I completely cut out alcohol and caffeine in any form out of my diet and… I feel amazing.
bigelow tea ginger honey plus zinc and tums antacid works for symptoms
I've been loving the effects of drinking <u>nettle and spearmint tea</u>[40] regularly.
I started drinking <u>raspberry leaf tea</u>[41] the week before my period and notice a much lighter cycle and no cramps.
I have a tea blend called Raspberry Meadows from <u>a small business</u>[42] where I used to live. It seems to help all my menstrual and premenstrual symptoms, even insomnia.

As much sunlight as possible
I got a road bike recently and have been biking around for hours.
I've been focusing on keeping my step count at over 10,000 a day (on average) and it has helped so much with symptoms.
Try a bike! Or rollerskating! Something fun! I skate and the favt that it is just pure FUN makes it so mu h easier to do it more often.

---

37 https://www.reddit.com/r/PMDDpartners/about/wiki/index/personalsuccess/
38 https://www.amazon.com/s?k=positive+pickle
39 http://www.reddit.com/r/PMDD/comments/1n268s3
40 http://www.reddit.com/r/PMDD/comments/1mq2miy
41 http://www.bbcgoodfood.com/health/nutrition/top-9-health-benefits-of-raspberry-leaf-tea
42 https://grandaddywillow.com/products/raspberry-meadows

My gp told me that 10,000 steps a day should have similar effect as antidepressant. Walking has also been a game changer to my symptoms, even if it's just a few minutes of walking.
trying to get 4k steps a day and stairmaster 4 times a week. omg.. omg omg.

I started using Anna's Wild Yam cream…wow it really was truly gorgeous to have a period sneak up on you.
This is the first time in over 25 years that I have had zero symptoms.
The two supplements that I took together were, WILD YAM CREAM (1 tsp 2x day under arms) and VITAMIN D, A AND K FORMULA (5 drops in AM). The vitamin D,A,K blend seemed to really have a good effect for me.

Editors note: See this post[43] about wild yam root. If it helps that is great but consult your doctor as there are a host of issues.

Serenol by Bonafide[44] (This is the most helpful one that was recommended by my gyno.)
So I have been on it for 6 months now and it's the first time I don't know when my period is coming because I'm not a monster and I don't hate everyone.
I also started taking Serenol (a supplement) and my period is much more regulated and I haven't had bad PMS in about 3 months!

Mostly I'm getting in the water and moving continuously for 30-60 minutes, then sitting in the hot tub for a bit. Something about being in the water makes me calm way way down and feel like I can handle life a little better.
Water is sorta like thunder vests for dogs. It's uniform deep pressure!
I just want to share my experience that the Wim Hof method (cold plunge) has me feeling better than I have in years.
Cold showers - I don't do them all the time, but when I do, my day just feels better.

I recently got a weighted blanket and although I have only used it for one cycle I haven't woken up in a panic/racing heartbeat/sweaty since using it. My luteal dreams are still odd/weird, but I don't encounter distressing dreams as often.

I have had 6 TMS treatments, and my rage was actually able to be managed this week.
I'm still not 100% prob 70% but before TMS I had deep deep scary depression

Editors Note: Transcranial Magnetic Stimulation is more commonly used for, and FDA approved for, Major Depressive Disorder.

---

43 https://www.reddit.com/r/PMDD/comments/1evbphs
44 http://www.reddit.com/r/PMDD/comments/1fmk92d

The Last Desperate Flail

I laid down and listened to some ASMR Reiki YouTubes by Healing by Sirena and
    wouldn't you know, they lulled me to sleep.
Lune inate has great videos too!
I love ediyamsr! Her voice is so soothing

---

testing your <u>free testosterone</u>[45] really can make a difference.
Also weight lifting gives you a natural testosterone boost so you might want to
    incorporate that as well.
I've been on testosterone for the last year due to low levels of T. It definitely helped
    with all my most difficult symptoms.
there's <u>some info I found recently</u>[46] that says anything under 25 for a woman in her
    childbearing years is actually low.

100mg b6. Also adding a calcium and magnesium during that week.
<u>B6 fixed my pmdd</u>.[47]
Bonus points for a complex. Most women are deficient in b vitamins.
I've taken vit d and b12 for about 4 months and the last three have been symptom
    free!
So I found a liquid vitamin with b6 and magnesium glysinate. It's been three weeks
    now and my anxiety has gotten so so much better.
B vitamins tend to help with boosting mood and energy. Magnesium helps with
    improving anxiety and sleep
Morning: Vit D -50 mcg Calcium (without the D) -500 mg Digestive probiotic Night:
    magnesium glycinate -400
Yeaaaah my doc instantly recommended B12 when I came in suspecting PMDD.

Calcium drops during luteal for everybody, so increasing supply helps a lot of people.
Calcium+vitamin d and magnesium
Vitamin D supplement. Vitamin D3+k2 to be exact
she said first to try taking a <u>calcium supplement</u>[48] during luteal and see how it
    went...it helped SO MUCH. I started 1500mg calcium few weeks before my luteal
    phase. No drama or brainfog, no ruminating or rage.
This is my 2nd month using coconut water for symptoms and every time I drink it they
    disappear. I did some research and apparently the body depletes magnesium,
    potassium, and calcium during this time of the month.

Editors Note: Vitamin K helps all the other vitamins get absorbed. Vitamin D helps
    calcium be absorbed. If you are deficient in Vitamin D calcium absorbtion will be
    blocked. Calcium is the only supplement specifically recommended by The
    American College of Obstetricians and Gynocologists for treating PMDD.
    Calcium, in turn, blocks absorbtion of magnesium so take your magnesium
    separately. Too much calcium can give you kidney stones. It's always something.

---

45 http://www.reddit.com/r/PMDD/comments/1n5o3vd
46 http://www.healthline.com/health/low-testosterone-in-women#treatments
47 http://www.reddit.com/r/PMDD/comments/1blagxj/comment/kw41jsc
48 http://www.reddit.com/r/PMDD/comments/1lgh1ot

Magnesium supplements helped me, and doing as much as i can physically during the good weeks. THC helps a lot.
Magnesium and primrose oil have also helped... oh and no coffee.
There are different types of magnesium and they don't all have the same function. So I take a multimagnesium that mixes 5 of them.
I tried ashwaganda with magnesium as recommended by someone on this subreddit. I have officially completed a whole cycle while on the supplement and it has changed my life.
Magnesium bisglycinate is more effective than Magnesium oxide!
dont hesitate to take glycinate magnesium also, it helps with irritability and anxiety

Evening primrose oil is a supplement that was recommended by my OBGYN. Progesterone cream was also recommended.

I started taking Sam E towards the end of my period last month, and here I am on Day 23 and have had very little to no emotional symptoms.

low doses of lithium oxolate[49] are sometimes very effective also as it's more bioavailable, and it's available OTC and not expensive

Took lysine[50] for a cold sore and noticed I barely felt any PMDD symptoms this month.

I love saffron. Wipes out 90% of my symptoms! Saffron helped my depression and focus too.

It feels like I'm experiencing normal PMS now, instead of the extreme feelings of wanting to ruin my life or die. Is anyone else taking lion's mane?

Try Pickle Juice[51] ... I don't know how it works, but it worked! Tears just stopped!
I thought the pickle juice was just for cramps but if it works for crying too then bless.
Pickle juice[52] = balancing potassium and sodium. Actually not that wild of a theory

CBD has changed my life and has effectively replaced lorazepam for me
CBD for the win. It's the only thing I do differently and everything is different.
Have you tried cannabis? Only thing that has successfully helped my rage.

---

49 http://www.reddit.com/r/PMDD/comments/1fcehix
50 http://www.reddit.com/r/PMDD/comments/1mg5760
51 http://www.reddit.com/r/PMDD/comments/1h2wnzf
52 http://www.reddit.com/r/PMDD/comments/1gti3rl

The Last Desperate Flail

I do a 50mg gummy (with 2mg THC) each day, cut in half. I take one half in the
morning and the other in the late afternoon. Maybe another half right before bed
if needed. I no longer take anything else (was using Yaz and various vitamins).
I'll take it forever.

I just started a krill oil supplement and evening primrose oil, and they have really kept
my mood out of the black. I still get mad and shit but I don't want to die, and
that's like.... fucking great.

I take L-Tryptophan[53] this cycle for the first time. 500-1000mg per day. I am on day
22 and normally hell would break loose. But I am feeling very good.
I have a rage issue and SI during luteal for 15 years now. I read about tryptophan[54]
and started taking it. I have just felt like a NORMAL person this whole cycle.
Incorporate foods high in tryptophan[55] (nuts, seeds, poultry, shellfish, oats). The
more the better.
One of the most bioavailable dietary forms of tryptophan is organic whey protein
concentrate[56], not isolate.

Editors Note: Tryptophan helps your body produce serotonin. If you are already on an
SSRI making more serotonin could increase your risk of developing serotonin
syndrom (too much serotonin). Obviously Thanksgiving dinner is okay but don't
go crazy. Talk to your doctor.

I started taking 5htp 100mg[57] in the morning about a week before my period and I
had ZERO PMDD symptoms.
happy to report that I am two months free[58] from crippling anxiety and suicidal
ideation!
The 5HTP I use is Natural Factors Time Release (I found, after trying 6 brands, that
the time release is critical).
ive been taking 5-HTP everyday for about two months now and it has helped ALOT.

Editors Note: Same as above. If you are already on an SSRI taking 5HTP could
increase your risk of developing serotonin syndrom (too much serotonin). Talk to
your doctor.

Taking your iron every other day instead of everyday will greatly diminish side effects
(this helps so much) For me i take ferrous gluconate 325, every other day. I wash
it down with a 100% vitamin C juice (usually cranberry)

---

53 http://www.reddit.com/r/PMDD/comments/1hdz6hp
54 http://www.reddit.com/r/PMDD/comments/1hdi30f
55 http://www.reddit.com/r/PMDD/comments/1dgjq30
56 http://www.reddit.com/r/PMDD/comments/1l8cvk7
57 http://www.reddit.com/r/PMDD/comments/1coosf5
58 http://www.reddit.com/r/PMDD/comments/u0as1m

For me correcting low ferritin[59] has almost completely eliminated my PMDD and debilitating periods.
Beef organ[60] supplements seem to help me!

I've never tried vitamin C supplements until this last month. I heard it could help - and I'm telling you - symptoms decreased by 80%. I'm shocked.
Who would've thought something so simple as a vitamin C pill would make such a difference. I'm so happy and relieved right now truly.
I remember reading one of the books about hormones and my main takeaway was that vitamin C and D are the first ones to supplement because they have kind of a chain reaction to the rest of the hormones.
I was taking large doses of Vitamin C[61] for immunity boost ... By that night, I was COMPLETELY NORMAL.
No techniques[62] but I take large doses of vitamin c and haven't experienced PMDD since.
5000 mg of vitamin c daily during PMDD days. I haven't experienced any PMDD symptoms since I started

---

For my current cycle I have used an estrogen patch ... and the past few days have felt entirely manageable.

Eating enough throughout the day (especially protein and hella healthy fats!!!)
Now I eat animal protein with every meal. I would say the biggest change though was going from never eating red meat to eating it at least 3-5 times a week.
I'll probably get downvoted but: the carnivore diet healed me.
protein protein protein![63]
Prioritizing eating whole foods during hell week. Meal prepping a few days before disaster strikes.
I decided I would try a low histamine diet during my luteal phase and something worked. I had no symptoms AT ALL.
we need more carbs (sweet potatoes, chick peas, butternut squash, apples, bananas, pumpkin seeds ext...), because progesterone needs glucose to function properly.
insanely restrictive diet[64] for two weeks and it totally reset my endocrine system.

Editors Note: Protein contains tryptophan which helps your body produce serotonin. If you are on an SSRI talk to your doctor about the risk of serotonin syndrom. The ketogegnic diet severely restricts sugar intake (none) to starve bad bacteria in the gut. Is not for everyone, talk to your doctor.

I tried about four rounds of acupuncture, and just saw a complete change on my last cycle.

59 http://www.reddit.com/r/PMDD/comments/1lgse60/comment/mz21qqw
60 http://www.reddit.com/r/PMDD/comments/1m2atud/comment/n3nnc2s
61 http://www.reddit.com/r/PMDDpartners/comments/1gl06n0
62 http://www.reddit.com/r/PMDD/comments/1kdibaj
63 http://www.reddit.com/r/PMDD/comments/1k4sbr5
64 http://www.reddit.com/r/PMDDpartners/comments/1l7vtml

The Last Desperate Flail

Hi all after trying everything under the sun, it seems that acupuncture is doing the trick.
YES!! Acupuncture has helped me immensely with regulating my hormones and thereafter, my pmdd!!
I tried acupuncture because I had nothing to lose and now I am able to feel happy in my luteal phase and I don't have any SI.
The only, only, only thing that has ever helped me is a really good acupuncturist[65]
2nd round of treatment[66] and it's been life changing so far.
what i love about Traditional Chinese Medicine[67] is that they work on finding the root cause
ELIX. It's traditional Chinese herbs that help for periods. I've used it six cycles now. This one I had the least cramps I've ever had in my whole life.
Idk traditional Chinese herbs feel it's not just masking the symptom but healing. It's made my pmdd go from like a 10 to a 5. This cycle I felt like a normal pmsing woman.
I tried taking Free and Easy Wanderer Plus (it's a traditional Chinese herbal remedy) every day for a few months and it did help a ton with my physical symptoms.

I just visited my local health store and they gave me a tincture of Passion Flower. I put it in my water a few hours ago and, wow. It helps a LOT.
Passionflower tastes like "the earth" 😋 but calms me down, or chills me out.
My naturopath suggested I use passionflower for moments when I'm really overwhelmed … and it has helped A LOT. It effectively stops the thought spiral and calms me down.

Alani nu balance supplement. Ive been taking it since January 2019 and it reduces my symptoms by 80%.

Vitex - saving my life tbh Vestura Vitamin d3 & k Magnesium Multi vitamin
Vitex/dim supplement called femgaurd plus balance

Editors Note: For some Vitex/dim has the opposite effect[68] you would hope for, so pay attention.

Chaste tree berry
Agnus castus / chaste berry daily through luteal phase
I finally decided to give chaste berry a shot … and it's literally changing my life.
chaste berry + B6, B12, magnesium, calcium, omega-3.

I ordered Jubilance because I was desperate…and it changed everything. I feel like a completely different person. Not just the hell week before my period, but all month.

65 http://www.reddit.com/r/PMDD/comments/1kg1wdn/comment/mqviqhu
66 http://www.reddit.com/r/PMDD/comments/1l4s4zo
67 http://www.reddit.com/r/PMDD/comments/1m5ivul
68 http://www.reddit.com/r/PMDD/comments/1ivvlp3

The supplement Jubilance aka oxaloacetate works magic for me.
I can now head [migraines] off if I take extra Jubilance, along with extra magnesium,
CoQ10, zinc, and vitamin D.

I've been taking NAC[69] for a couple months now (N-Acetyl Cysteine) and it helps
calm a lot of the emotional pain and stress down for me in general but especially
during luteal.

Keto diet. I read Brain Energy by Dr Chris Palmer (Harvard psychiatrist), was so
impressed that he mentioned PMDD in his book that i figured what the heck, I'll
give this a shot. It's the first diet I've been able to stick to in a decade AND it's
helping my anxiety and PMDD!

Irritable moods: So far I've found strong chocolate like 74%-86% cacao and for some
reason oatmeal cream pies help.
Yes!!! Twinnings Lemon & Ginger tea, dark dark dark chocolate, spinach salads,
hydration, all my go to's as well.
I'll add Yogi Immune + Stress tea with ashwagandha.
Lavender teas. Nature, exercise and meditation as consistently as possible :)

I started taking Ashwaghanda every morning. For the past two months I have been
symptom free.
After doing much research on this very sub, I immediately purchased ashwagandha
and vitamin d3 & k2. I noticed immediate change in my mood after consuming
ashwa (KSM66). I only take it during luteal phase.
Holy crap, it helped me SO MUCH[70]. About a half hour after taking it I felt calmer and
happier, more like myself.

Two months ago I've had enough and decided to try meditating hardcore. Not just 5
or 10 minutes a day but a grueling 1 hour a day meditation regimen. Then luteal
hit [and] there was no sign of rage or panic attacks…

I started mircodosing psilocybin[71]. This shit was life changing on a number of
levels.
what I love about mushrooms is that I can take them on an as-needed basis and it
functions much like an antidepressant.

Hi all after trying everything under the sun, it seems that acupuncture[72] is doing the
trick.

69 http://www.reddit.com/r/PMDD/comments/1lndwtq
70 http://www.reddit.com/r/PMDD/comments/1jlv3zz
71 http://www.reddit.com/r/PMDD/comments/1izje7r
72 http://www.reddit.com/r/PMDD/comments/1csqbaj

The Last Desperate Flail

Acupuncture has been a lifesaver for me.
Yes! PMDD is the reason my mom found acupuncture in the first place! ...
    acupuncture + herbs really helped me eliminate my symptoms for a long time.
It probably saved my life. I found a dr of Chinese medicine that specialised in
    women's health and hormone health.
acupuncture once a month on the same day/close to same day. It helps regulates
    things and I notice my PMDD is way more manageable.
I started acupuncture[73] for PMDD this cycle. They also gave me some Xiao Yao San
    tablets ... it's just hit me that my luteal phase has been...really good?
acupuncture combined with Traditional Chinese Medicine and supplements has
    removed 95% of my symptoms.

L-Theanine[74] w/ GABA and B-complex along w eating enough & working out
L-theanine + lemon balm is really good Helps with anxiety, chills you out
L-theanine, lemon balm and b-complex vitamins are a must.
L- Theanine[75]...started taking 200mg a day- only the week to ten days before my
    period ... I was completely symptom free!

I saw someone mention the clean marine vitamins. They're really expensive though
    so I got the 3 main things separately for a third the price and tried those: omega
    complex (3,6,9), d 1000, and b6.

Magnesium glycinate before bed
Magnesium, psyllium husk, red raspberry leaf tea, plenty of seeds (chia, hemp, flax,
    etc.)
I've had chronic diarrhoea ... found psyllium husk[76] recommend ... almost
    unbelievably for me, period is due in two days and I've had no major mood
    swings, I'm functioning well. I was energised yesterday and went on a 4hr hike.
i recommend at least trying it and seeing how your body responds! i was shocked to
    notice a change[77] even in a short period.

Editors Note: most seeds contain tryptophan which helps your body produce
    serotonin. If you are on an SSRI talk to your doctor about the risk of serotonin
    syndrom. Additional fiber can help round up and expel excess estrogen.

I've been taking my Ritual Womens Multi Vitamin every day this cycle, and I'm 5 days
    from bleed with literally no symptoms. That tagged with, my Green Drink which is
    Garden of life brand.

Antihistamines daily through luteal phase.

73 http://www.reddit.com/r/PMDD/comments/1izjqzo
74 http://www.reddit.com/r/PMDD/comments/1f9vi8d
75 http://www.reddit.com/r/PMDD/comments/1krxg1z
76 http://www.reddit.com/r/PMDD/comments/1m9t2eg
77 http://www.reddit.com/r/PMDD/comments/1md8xk8

I saw someone mentioning histamine as one of the contributing factors to PMDD. I took antihistamine for almost a month and it worked for me.

Editors Note: If antihistamines help with your PMDD symptoms get checked for Mast Cell Activation Syndrome (MCAS).

Prozac, lamictal, vitamin d, magnesium, heavy weight training 5x a week, 20 min cardio 3-4x a week, social circle, living with my best friend.
Lamictal and DBT skills. The Lamictal makes it easier to use the skills and using the skills increases my quality of life, so they complement each other very nicely.
The right combo of meds. Lamictal + Abilify (actually now Rexulti) has taken symptoms from 10/10 literally debilitating with family begging me to go to hospital down to 2/10 mildly annoying

---

I've decided that during luteal i'm going to treat myself as if I have BPD[78], and do all the DBT skills one would for borderline. I also doubled my prozac dose.

SuperYou by Moon Juice. its specifically made for stress and they're vegan/cruelty-free/etc. they are just supplement capsules (and tbh they taste awful) but the results for me were noticeable almost immediately.

Focusmate to help me get work done when I'm fatigued and have brain fog.

But Wait! There's More!

Here is an entire post about AI that reads like a Ronco ad.[79] Also try Pi.ai if you're between therapists at the moment.

Here is an entire thread of more things that might help[80].

And another[81]. And another[82]. And another[83].

If you have tried something not on the list, that worked well, let the mods know.

For example: Ketamine IV, low dose ketamine, microdosing[84], peyote, floating, hypnotherapy, Cat rescue, slam poetry, trampoline, …

---

78 http://www.reddit.com/r/PMDD/comments/1i1xuti
79 http://www.reddit.com/r/PMDD/comments/1dbzn1y
80 http://www.reddit.com/r/PMDD/comments/1e1854d
81 http://www.reddit.com/r/PMDD/comments/1fqkpbq
82 http://www.reddit.com/r/PMDD/comments/1gil801
83 http://www.reddit.com/r/PMDD/comments/1iathbj
84 http://www.reddit.com/r/microdosing/comments/14o26ur

Three Simple Steps for Managing Anger

NOTICE: Be alert, aware of your signals of anger, then…

SEPARATE & CALM DOWN: get away from events, triggers, persons, and offensive factors by physically and mentally leaving.

PLAN & ASSERT: Think through what to say or do. Choose a respectful and appropriate response that will attack the problem, not the person. Ask if the other person is ready. When the time is right, discuss it calmly to find solutions.

What is your goal? What motivated you to seek help?

SIGNALS: What are triggers and responses in you that warn you are getting frustrated, irritated, or angry: Sensations, body language, voice, words, situations?

1.

2.

3.

4.

5.

6.

7.

8.

Read these signals at least once a day for at least one month to remember them and recognize them when they occur.

During the time out when you are separated, what will you do to calm down so you can think well again with all of your intelligence and problem-solving abilities (relaxation, activities, physical exercise, etc.)?

I will _

After I'm calm, I think, "So, why am I angry and how do I say what I feel?"

By Brian Floyd Bubeck – included by permission.

When you are able to think clearly again, and able to anticipate and care about the results of your choices again, ask yourself...

What needs, concerns, interests, or values do I care about in this situation?
How are those needs, concerns, interests, or values threatened?
Is this an observed and actual threat or just one I suspect or interpret?
If it is not actual or observed at this time, how likely is it to happen?

If the threat to your values, interests, plans, expectations or goals is an actual observed reality, or very likely to happen, and if your expectations were realistic, your anger is rational. If you are in an ongoing relationship with the person who presents this trouble, then assertiveness is the reliable way to let go of your anger.

However, though it is healthy to be assertive, it is not always safe or always legal. Do not speak or act assertively if you believe it could result in harm or danger to anyone, including yourself.

Don't risk assertiveness with people who have have a history of violence toward other people. Don't express anger assertively if you risk catastrophic losses (job, income) or lawsuits. Don't express assertively if you believe you could receive legal consequences like being charged with a crime. In these situations, you need to get away from the threatening situation or people and seek protection and help. Before taking such risks seek expert medical, legal, and mental health advice to manage risks.

But if we are realistic about it, most of the situations that make us angry do not come with those risks. So we need to be assertive.

Plan and rehearse how you will say it:

I statements (Not You Statements) are a proven method of assertive communication that are the most successful method yet developed. Rehearse this in time out:

I feel ________________(state a feeling word like angry, sad, afraid, etc.)

When you ___________(objectively describe the current or recent event, not patterns or personality descriptions or absolutes like always and never.)

Because ____________(describe your perception of the threat to your values, interests, and concerns, or your reasons for the feelings.)

And what I want is_____(the specific observable action, behavior or change that would meet the need, concern, value, or interest).

By Brian Floyd Bubeck – included by permission.

The Last Desperate Flail

Ask the other person if they are ready to hear your concerns, and wait for them to be calm, respectful, and ready before you discuss it. A good test is can you say out loud your I statement without pausing long periods of time, and it sounds nice when you say it. But the second test is needed too. Are you ready to listen to a view that you disagree with, and still respect and validate that view and those concerns? If not, wait till you are ready for both. But don't put it off or avoid the conversation. If you try, you can get calm and be prepared to give respect. So somewhere between a half hour and 24 hours after the conflict, for most ordinary conflicts you can talk it out. A life altering tragic event may need longer time to get ready, but not every day conflicts.

When you are ready, ask the other person if they are calm and ready to talk it out respectfully, taking turns, and respecting each other's concerns and different views. Monitoring your tone and calm/respectful speech and volume with I Statements, and Active Listening. Here is the combined script for both speaker and listener roles:

I feel_____________________(state a feeling word like angry, sad, afraid, etc.)

When you ________________(objectively describe the current or recent event, not patterns or personality descriptions or absolutes like always and never.)

Because ________________(describe your perception of the threat to your values, interests, and concerns, or your reasons for the feelings.)

And what I want is _________(the specific observable action, behavior or change that would meet the need, concern, value, or interest).

If I heard you right, you feel _________________________________
When I ____
Because ____
And what you want is ______________________________________
Do you feel understood? If no, try speaker and listener parts again.

Is there more? (if yes, go through another speaker and listener exchange)

Then when the speaker feels understood about that particular event, the roles are switched, and the speaker becomes the active listener, and the listener becomes the next speaker saying their own I statement.

Thank you for your efforts to improve your relationships and your mood and mental health with that.

By Brian Floyd Bubeck – included by permission.

Symptom Tracker

PREMENSTRUAL SYMPTOM TRACKER
(DAILY RECORD OF SEVERITY OF PROBLEMS)

Name:

Month:

INSTRUCTIONS

Print off as many copies as you need to complete a **full two months** worth of tracking. Begin tracking your premenstrual symptoms with this chart today. Fill it out **daily** (preferably at the end of your day). Two full months of menstrual cycle charting will allow for a more accurate assessment.

Each evening note the degree to which you experienced each of the problems listed below. Put an "x" in the box which corresponds to the severity:

1 - not at all   **2 - minimal**   3 - mild   **4 - moderate**   5 - severe   **6 - extreme**

SYMPTOMS

	Enter day of the week (e.g. Monday = 'M') / Note any spotting by entering 'S' / Note menstrual bleeding by entering 'M' / Date (i.e. 1 = 1st of the month)
1.	Felt depressed, sad, "down,", or "blue" or felt hopeless; or felt worthless or guilty
2.	Felt anxious, tense, "keyed up" or "on edge"
3.	Had mood swings (i.e., suddenly feeling sad or tearful) or was sensitive to rejection or feelings were easily hurt
4.	Felt angry, or irritable
5.	Had less interest in usual activities (work, school, friends, hobbies)
6.	Had difficulty concentrating
7.	Felt lethargic, tired, or fatigued; or had lack of energy
8.	Had increased appetite or overate; or had cravings for specific foods
9.	Slept more, took naps, found it hard to get up when intended; or had trouble getting to sleep or staying asleep
10.	Felt overwhelmed or unable to cope; or felt out of control
11.	Had breast tenderness, breast swelling, bloated sensation, weight gain, headache, joint or muscle pain, or other physical symptoms

IMPACT

	At work, school, home, or in daily routine, at least one of the problems noted above caused reduction of production or efficiency
	At least one of the problems noted above caused avoidance of or less participation in hobbies or social activities
	At least one of the problems noted above interfered with relationships with others

https://www.iapmd.org/shop/p/iapmd-pmds-symptom-tracker

PREMENSTRUAL SYMPTOM TRACKER
(DAILY RECORD OF SEVERITY OF PROBLEMS)

Name:

Month:

INSTRUCTIONS

Print off as many copies as you need to complete a full **two months** worth of tracking. Begin tracking your premenstrual symptoms with this chart today. Fill it out **daily** (preferably at the end of your day). Two cycle charting will allow for a more accurate assessment.

Each evening note the degree to which you experienced each of the problems listed below. Put an "x" in the box which corresponds to the severity:

1 - not at all   **2 - minimal**   3 - mild   **4 - moderate**   5 - severe   6 - extreme

SYMPTOMS

		1	2	3	4	5	6	7	8	9	10	11	12	13	14	15	16	17	18	19	20	21	22	23	24	25	26	27	28	29	30	31
Enter day of the week (e.g. Monday = 'M')		s	s	m	t	w	t	f																									

Enter day of the week (e.g. Monday = 'M').
Note start of bleeding by entering 'S'.
Note menses ending by entering 'M'.
(i.e. 1 = 1st of the month)

1. Felt depressed, sad, "down,", or "blue" or hopeless; or felt worthless or guilty

2. Felt anxious, tense, "keyed up" or "on edge"

3. Had mood swings (e.g. suddenly feeling sad or tearful) or was sensitive to rejection or feelings were easily hurt

4. Felt angry, or irritable

5. Had less interest in usual activities (work, school, friends, hobbies)

6. Had difficulty concentrating

7. Felt lethargic, tired, or fatigued; or had lack of energy

8. Had increased appetite or overate; or had cravings for specific foods

9. Slept more, took naps, found it hard to get up when intended; or had trouble getting to sleep or staying asleep

10. Felt overwhelmed or unable to cope; or felt out of control

11. Had breast tenderness, breast swelling, bloated sensation, weight gain, headache, joint or muscle pain, or other physical symptoms

IMPACT

At work, school, home, or in daily routine, at least one of the problems noted above caused reduction of production of efficiency

At least one of the problems noted above caused avoidance of or less participation in hobbies or social activities

At least one of the problems noted above interfered with relationships with others

iapmd.org/steps-to-diagnosis for more information on gaining a PMD diagnosis

2021 © International Association For Premenstrual Disorders
Adapted from Jean Endicott, Ph.D. and Wilma Harrison, M.D. version

Other Resources

Books:

Aaron Kinghorn: Hope - A Guide to PMDD for Partners & Caregivers

Shalene Gupta: The Cycle - Confronting the Pain of Periods and PMDD

YouTube Channels:

My Therapist's a Witch: https://www.youtube.com/@elizabeth.ferreira/

PMDD with C: https://www.youtube.com/@PMDDwithC

Organizations:

IAPMD.org (International Association for Premenstrual Disorders)

The PMDD Project: https://thepmddproject.org/

Blogs:

The Belle Health Blog: https://bellehealth.co/blog/

PMDD Ventures: https://pmddventuresblog.wordpress.com/

Period/Symptom Trackers:

Belle: https://bellehealth.co/

Stardust: https://stardust.app/

Crisis Resources:

International crisis hotlines: helpguide.org/find-help

Acknowledgments

Members of the sub have all contributed even if just lurking. We post and comment to help each other, but also for those who just read and, hopefully, get what they need.

Most members are partners or family members of women with PMDD, but some sympathetic women who have PMDD themselves have also offered sage advice/support.

Reddit is anonymous by design and we have no wish to dox anyone.

Thanks to:

PadreDeBlas
HusbandofPMDD
dontwakethellama
TasteGlittering4459
Baloneous_V
MustyEssay
IndelibleScrapyard429
OkContext5658
Mugatu-Utagum
SophiaFalconePMDD
Infoseek456
doblador_de_tierra
Sorry-Story4498
Willing_Promise1508
Total_Personality952

stop_look_listen
WeakHaircut
Extension-Message-12
Far-Structure-6933
Lill1992
Icy_Resolution5282
GetTheLead_Out
FarReaction
0hh0n3y
Specific-Frame8833
donivan-floyd
Agitated_Ad9471
Remarkable-Banana512
JobAromatic7843
TurbidArtifact
Tubular_Jeeves126

The couples that make it

are the ones that can work together

against the common enemy.

You are the lion.

It can't escalate if you're not there.

She'll calm down a lot faster,
and have a lot less to regret later,
if you're not there.

Greyrocking is a survival strategy,
not a lifestyle choice.

Greyrock as long as it takes to leave,
leave as quickly as possible.

Whatever you do when you can't take it anymore ...
do that right away.

You're going to be wrong no matter what you do,
so you may as well do what's right.

As soon as you realize it is one of *those* conversations ...
Walk Away

It's not an endurance test or a feat of strength.
Walk Away.

Save your energy,
use it for something that makes a difference,
like making dinner.

Walk Away.
If she follows walk further, walk faster.

It takes two to tango but it only takes one to push and bait and
insult and berate and belittle and push some more until the
other person reacts and then claim it takes two to tango.